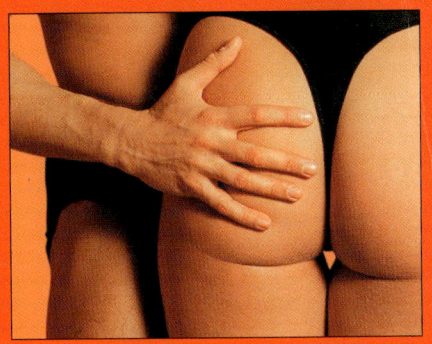

GREAT SEX SECRETS

ANNE HOOPER

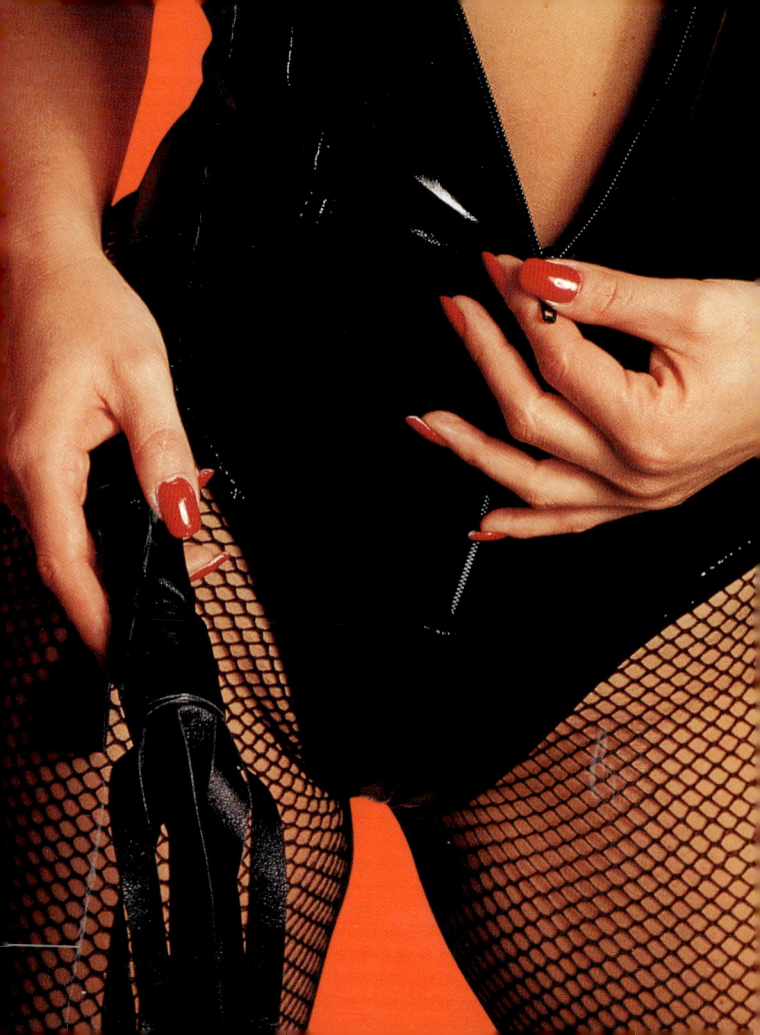

GREAT SEX SECRETS

ANNE HOOPER

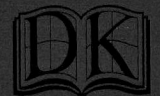

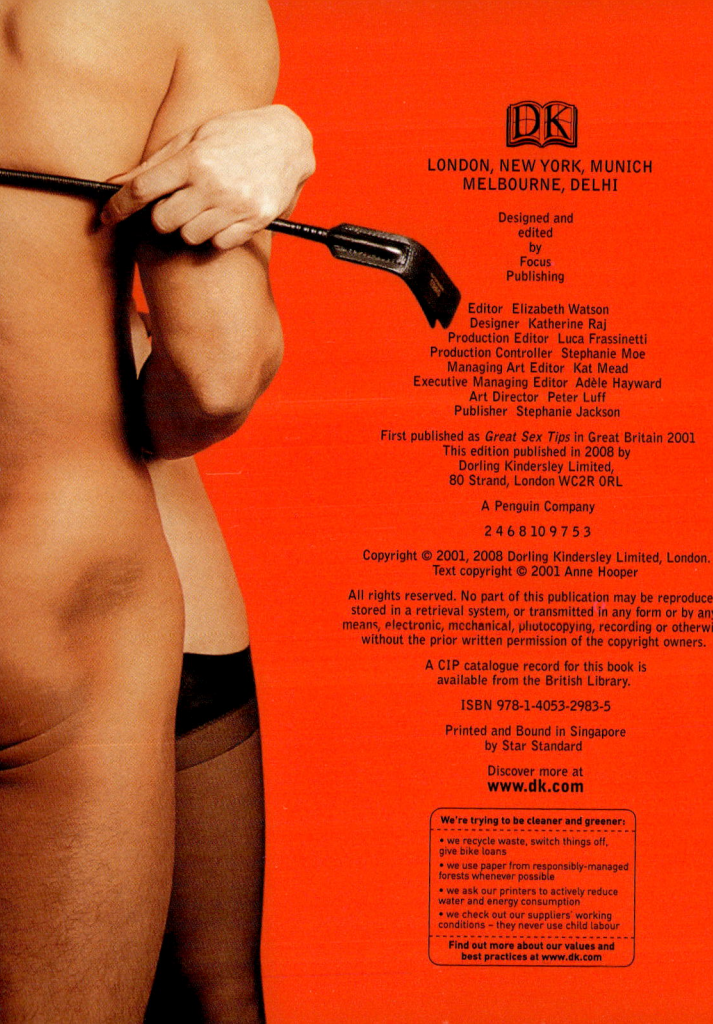

DK

LONDON, NEW YORK, MUNICH
MELBOURNE, DELHI

Designed and
edited
by
Focus
Publishing

Editor Elizabeth Watson
Designer Katherine Raj
Production Editor Luca Frassinetti
Production Controller Stephanie Moe
Managing Art Editor Kat Mead
Executive Managing Editor Adèle Hayward
Art Director Peter Luff
Publisher Stephanie Jackson

First published as *Great Sex Tips* in Great Britain 2001
This edition published in 2008 by
Dorling Kindersley Limited,
80 Strand, London WC2R 0RL

A Penguin Company

2 4 6 8 10 9 7 5 3

Copyright © 2001, 2008 Dorling Kindersley Limited, London.
Text copyright © 2001 Anne Hooper

All rights reserved. No part of this publication may be reproduced,
stored in a retrieval system, or transmitted in any form or by any
means, electronic, mechanical, photocopying, recording or otherwise,
without the prior written permission of the copyright owners.

A CIP catalogue record for this book is
available from the British Library.

ISBN 978-1-4053-2983-5

Printed and Bound in Singapore
by Star Standard

Discover more at
www.dk.com

We're trying to be cleaner and greener:

• we recycle waste, switch things off,
give bike loans

• we use paper from responsibly-managed
forests whenever possible

• we ask our printers to actively reduce
water and energy consumption

• we check out our suppliers' working
conditions – they never use child labour

**Find out more about our values and
best practices at www.dk.com**

CONTENTS

Introduction 6

Seduction 10
In the Mood 38
Loving Him 80
Loving Her 116
Erotic Toys 156
Sex Games 190

Index 236
Acknowledgements 240

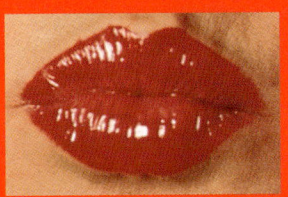

INTRODUCTION

INTRODUCTION

This little book of sex tips has been designed as a pillow book. It is colorful, saucy, something to keep by the side of the bed, something to dip into, something with which to entertain your lover. It is supposed to be fun. It is definitely not intended as a deadly serious sex manual. Sex is best fun when it's done with an open mind.

The value of **Great Sex Tips** is that it is chock-full with things to make your love life a little more lively. When I used to run groups for women with sex problems, one

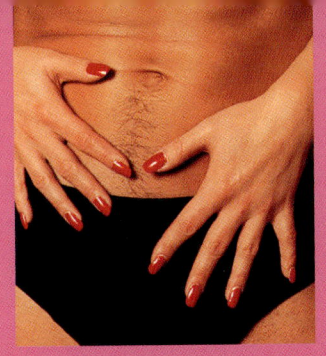

of the things they had great difficulty with was fun. It was almost as if "because it was sex it shouldn't be a game." And yet some of the best sex takes the form of games, or of dressing up.

Playing with food, of course, was another thing we were forbidden to do as small children. Perhaps that is why the combination of food and sex is so exciting to some lovers. It feels like doing two absolute "forbiddens" at the same time!

INTRODUCTION

Bath time for many innocents is a time of pure sensuality. The steam, the sweet smells, the slippery motion of a lover's hand sliding liquid soap down the length of the body ... We ALL want to be seduced! All men and women adore having attention focused physically at every inch of their yearning skin. Here are a few ideas how to tempt, tantalize, and torture.

Anne Hooper

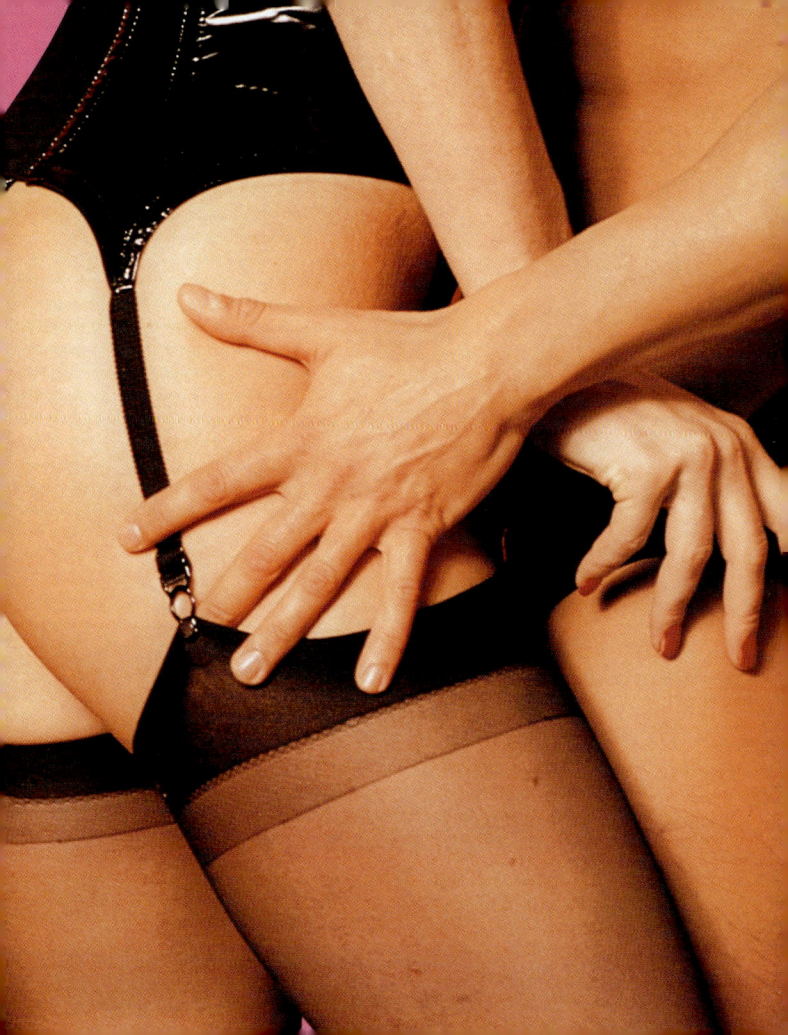

CHAPTER 1
SEDU

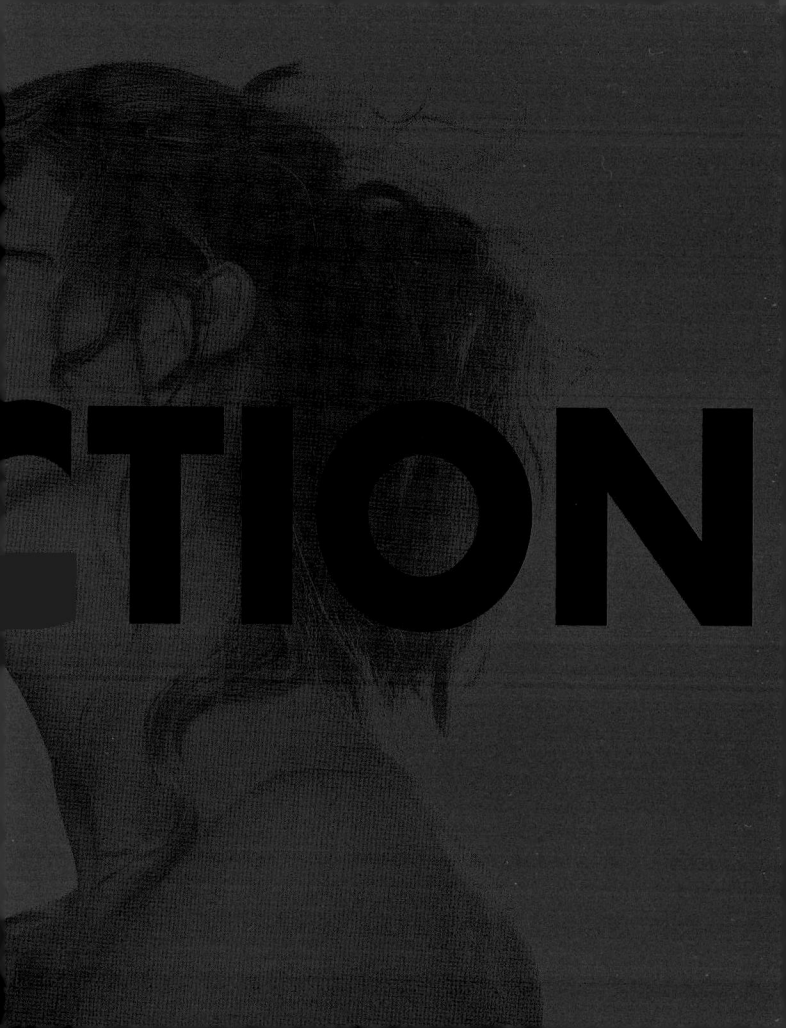

SEDUCTION

BE
HOT

❤ Men are turned on by what they see, so dress sexily, push back your shoulders, look your guy straight in the eye, and give him your most provocative smile.

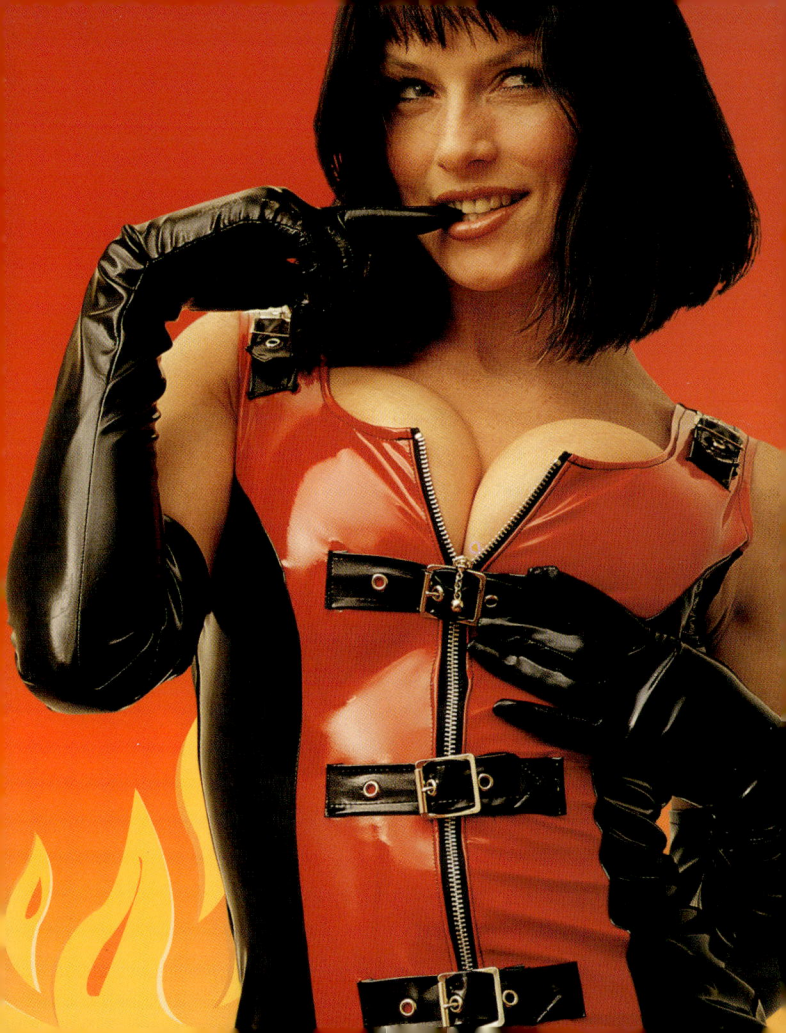

SEDUCTION

CHEMISTRY
LESSON

♥ Learn about pheromones, the chemicals that are produced by our bodies and that influence sexual responses in a mate. If you feel particularly horny around someone, chances are you're attracted to their pheromones.

♥ Smell your lover's t-shirt after they have worn it for a day, and see how it makes you feel.

SEDUCTION

❤ Enhance exposure to each other's pheromones by washing less.

❤ See what happens when you don't wear perfume or aftershave for a couple of days. Perfume blocks your pheromones.

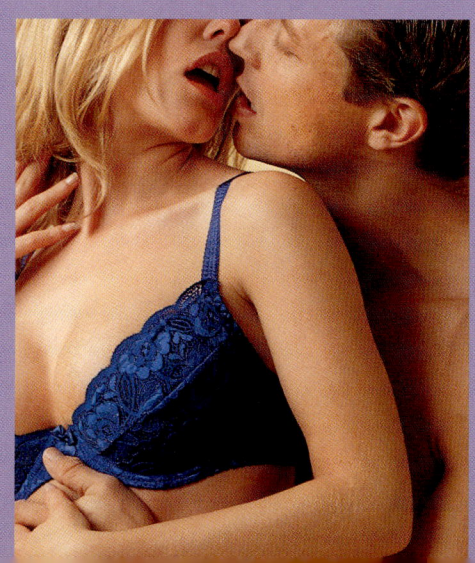

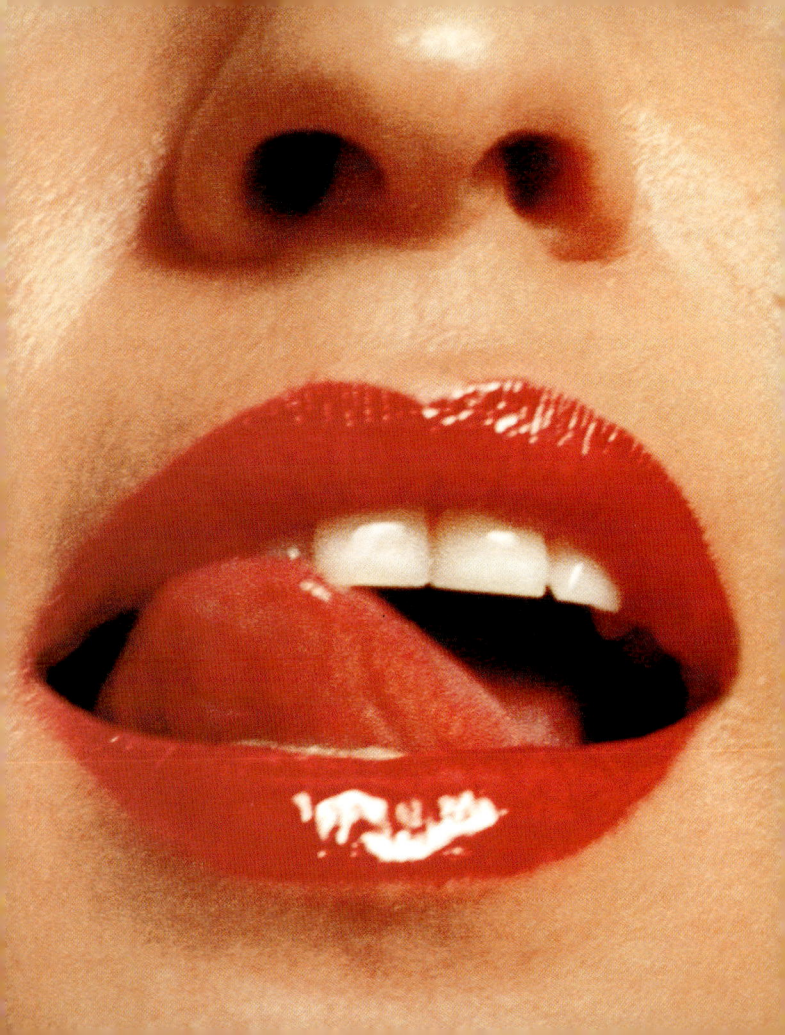

SEDUCTION

LUSCIOUS
LIPS

♥ Luscious lips do more to attract a mate than any other facial feature. Big red lips are a major attraction, so don't be afraid of using bold colors and lots of shiny lip gloss.

♥ If your lips are naturally small, smile – this stretches them and makes them look bigger and sexier.

SEDUCTION

SWEET
HEART

♥ Try some romantic role reversal. Send him flowers and champagne.

♥ Write each other an old-fashioned love letter and send it through the mail – even if you see each other every day.

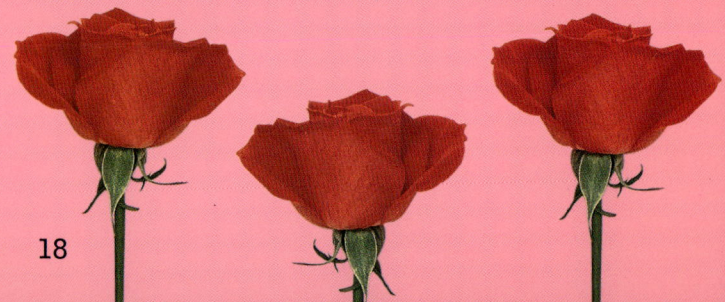

SEDUCTION

❤ Meet her from work when she's not expecting it.

❤ Go on romantic outings. Take him to a carnival or funfair, share some candy, and kiss passionately on the big wheel.

❤ Avoid romantic no-nos such as shabby underwear, hard-core porn, furry handcuffs, and unwashed bodies.

❤ Choose a romantic song together.

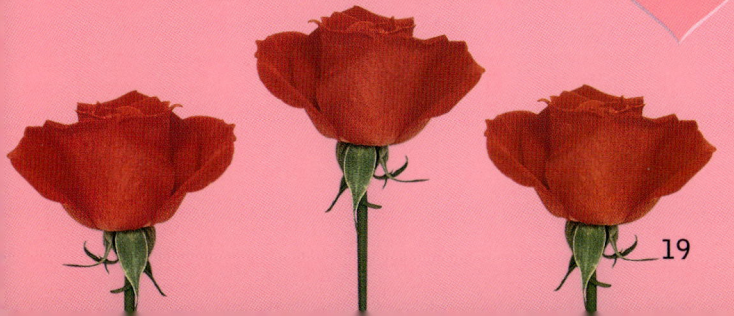

SEDUCTION

DRESSING
DOWN

❤ Women: rather than stripping naked for sex, leave on a few carefully chosen items of underwear, such as black lacy stockings and a garter.

❤ Men: strip down to some tight or silky boxer shorts that emphasize the shape of your buttocks.

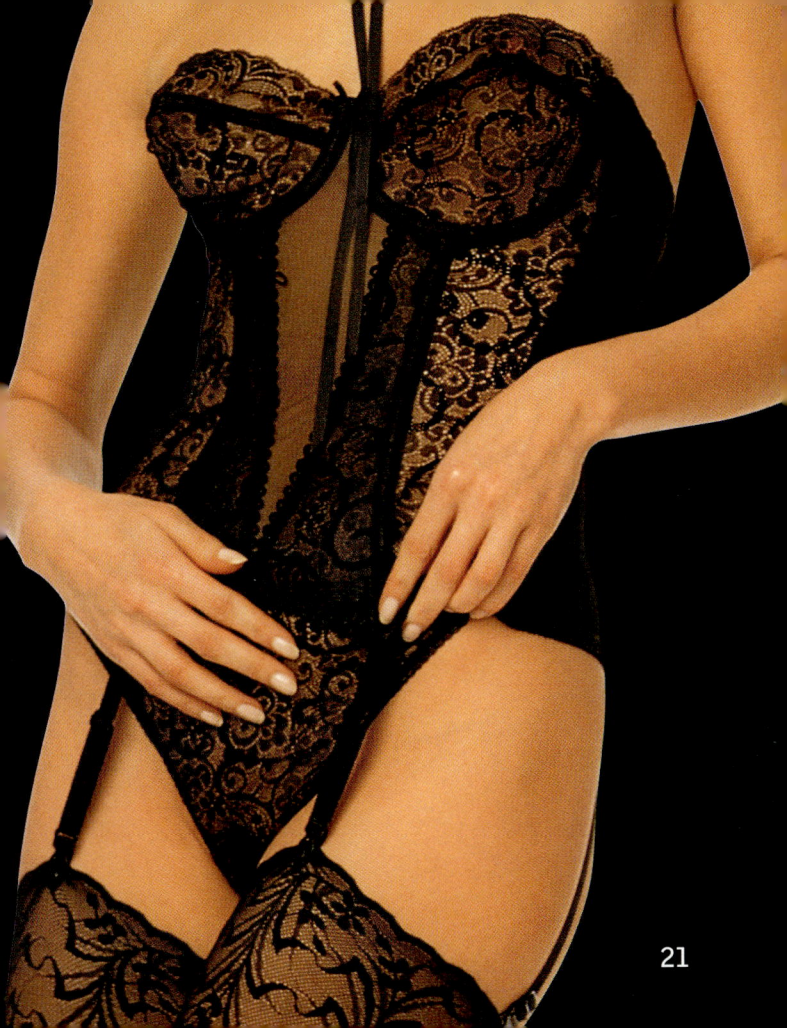

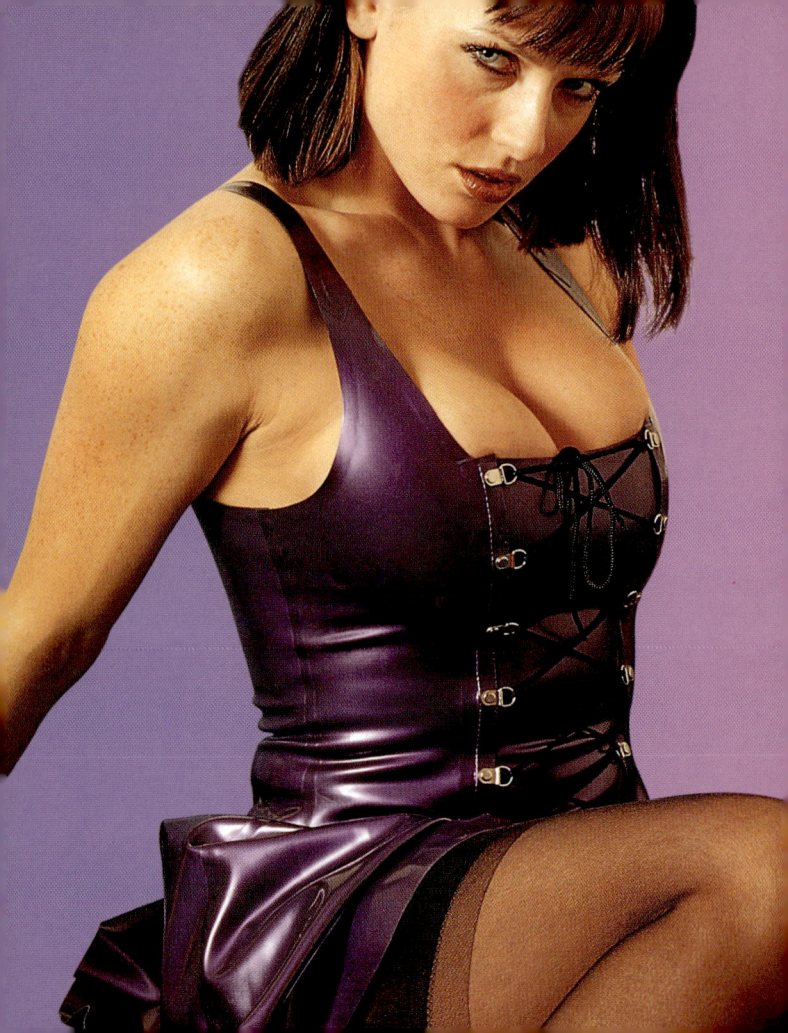

SEDUCTION

FLIRTING
FUN

❤ Women: lick your lips, move toward your man, and ensure that lots of silky leg is showing. As he shifts position, mirror his actions.

❤ Men: sit lower than her and gaze upward into her eyes. Tell her that she's the sexiest person you've met in years.

SEDUCTION

❤ Women: when you are sitting down, extend your arms along the back of the chair or sofa to show how open you are to his charms.

❤ Men: touch your partner lightly on the small of the back.

❤ Women: brush past him accidentally on purpose!

❤ Men: look her in the eye when she talks. Make her feel that you are interested in what she is saying.

❤ Women: listen carefully and ask him lots of questions.

SEDUCTION

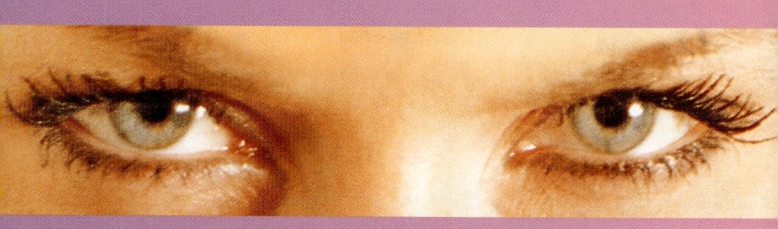

❤ Men: pay her lots of compliments.

❤ Women: get closer as you chat, so that you're almost but not quite touching.

❤ Men: hold back from doing anything overtly sexual too soon. You are just laying the groundwork for sexual attraction!

❤ Men and women: keep up close eye contact throughout – the eyes have it!

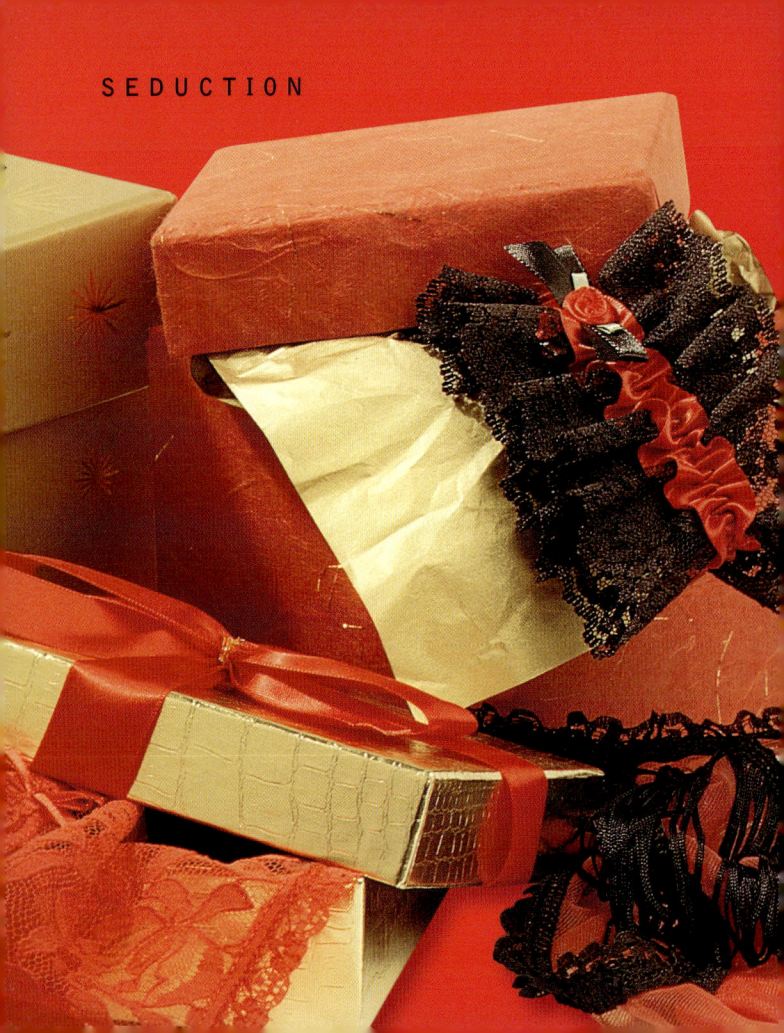

SEDUCTION

SAUCY
SURPRISES

♥ Everyone loves a surprise, and the saucier the better. When your relationship is heating up, send each other sexy books and suggestive cards. When it's truly on the boil, send champagne or exotic lingerie.

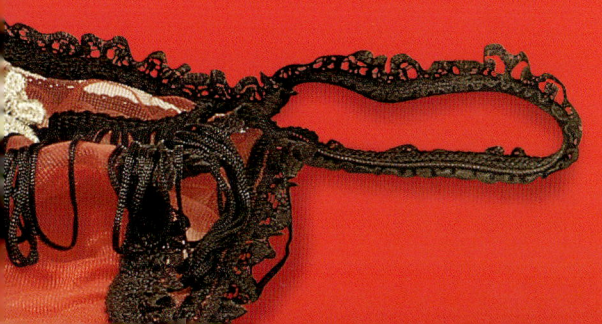

SEDUCTION

ROMANTIC
MEALS

❤ Make a meal visually gorgeous. Surround a bright red shellfish, such as lobster or crab, with brilliant green salad leaves. For dessert, create a platter of exotic fruits, beautifully cut and arranged in a pattern.

❤ Feed each other finger foods or spoonfuls of ice-cream.

❤ Lick your partner's sticky fingers.

SEDUCTION

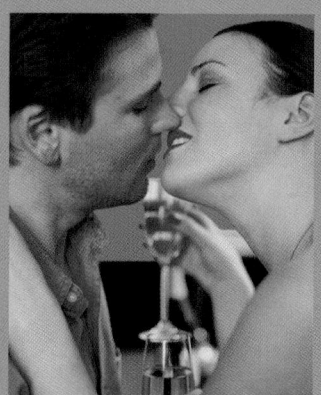

❤ Gaze at each other as you eat and play footsie under the table.

❤ Propose a toast to each other and to the evening ahead.

❤ Gnaw sexily on a chicken leg in front of your partner – in Tom Jones-style.

SEDUCTION

SEX
TOKEN

❤ Create a book of sex tokens: each one contains a sexual promise such as "I promise to pay the bearer one incredible sexual massage/a game of domination and submission/a dozen orgasms/an hour of sexual slavery."

❤ Tell her in advance when she can use a sex token and, for an extra-special treat, let her choose her favorite.

SEDUCTION

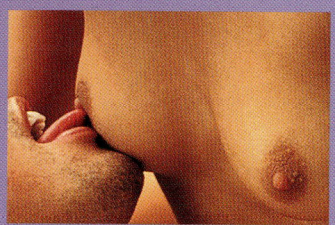

❤ Hide a sex token in his trouser pocket, under his pillow, in his briefcase, or in the glove compartment of his car. Write at the bottom: "To be redeemed as soon as we next meet."

❤ Make some extra-special sex tokens that explain in minute detail how you plan to seduce your partner from the very first touch to the last.

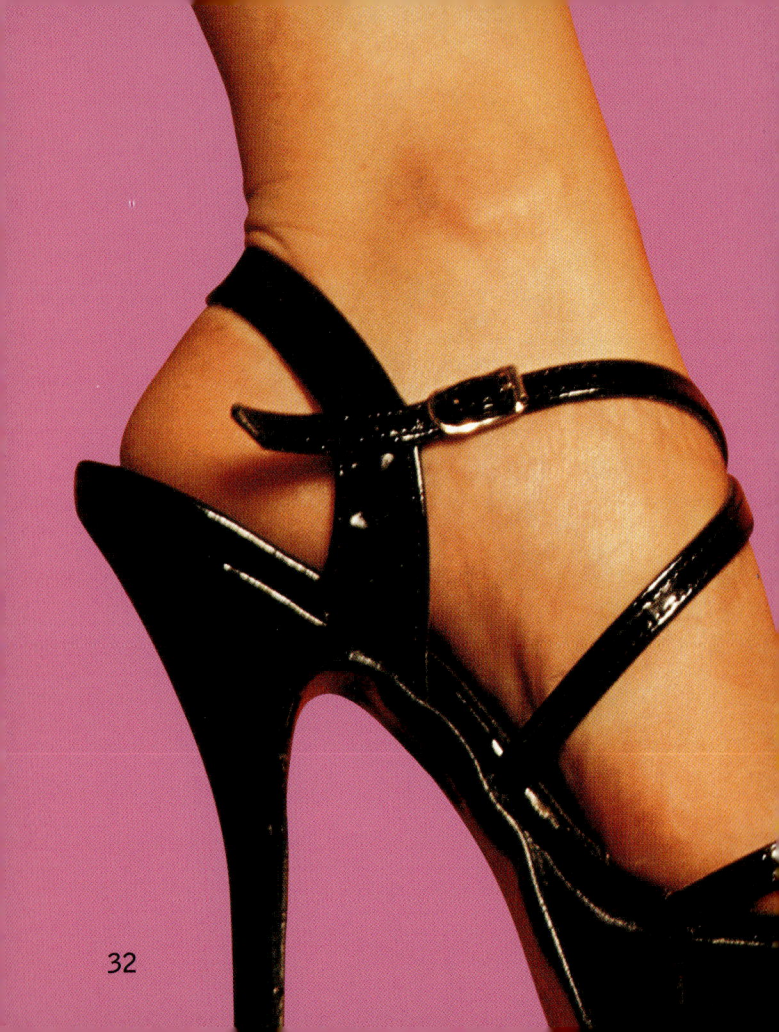

SEDUCTION

THE
LOOK

❤ The tighter your clothes, the longer your legs, and the higher your heels, the sexier you appear. But a word of caution: you should also dress so that you feel comfortable. Awkwardness shows.

❤ If your legs are on show, check that your skin is silky smooth and caressable.

SEDUCTION

TECH
TALK

❤ Leave flattering messages on your partner's voicemail.

❤ Have phone sex. Describe in graphic detail what you'd like to do to each other and what you're doing to yourself.

❤ Send your partner a text message just after you've parted to say you can't wait to meet up again.

SEDUCTION

❤ Exchange erotic emails with each other at work. Substitute code words for sex so that no-one else will understand.

❤ Send your partner an erotic greeting card by email: check out www.kinkycards.com.

❤ Email your partner with details of your chat room and arrange to meet there later.

❤ Send him a link for a website that sells sexy underwear and suggest he buys you a present.

❤ Buy webcams for your computers so that you can watch each other getting turned on as you chat or email.

SEDUCTION

TEMPTING
TORSO

❤ If you've got a tight and muscly torso, show it off to your lover. Walk around at home wearing black shorts.

❤ Cosmetics aren't just for women. Rub sweet-smelling oil or moisturizer into your skin – all over.

❤ Seduce her when you've just come out of the bathroom with a towel wrapped around your waist.

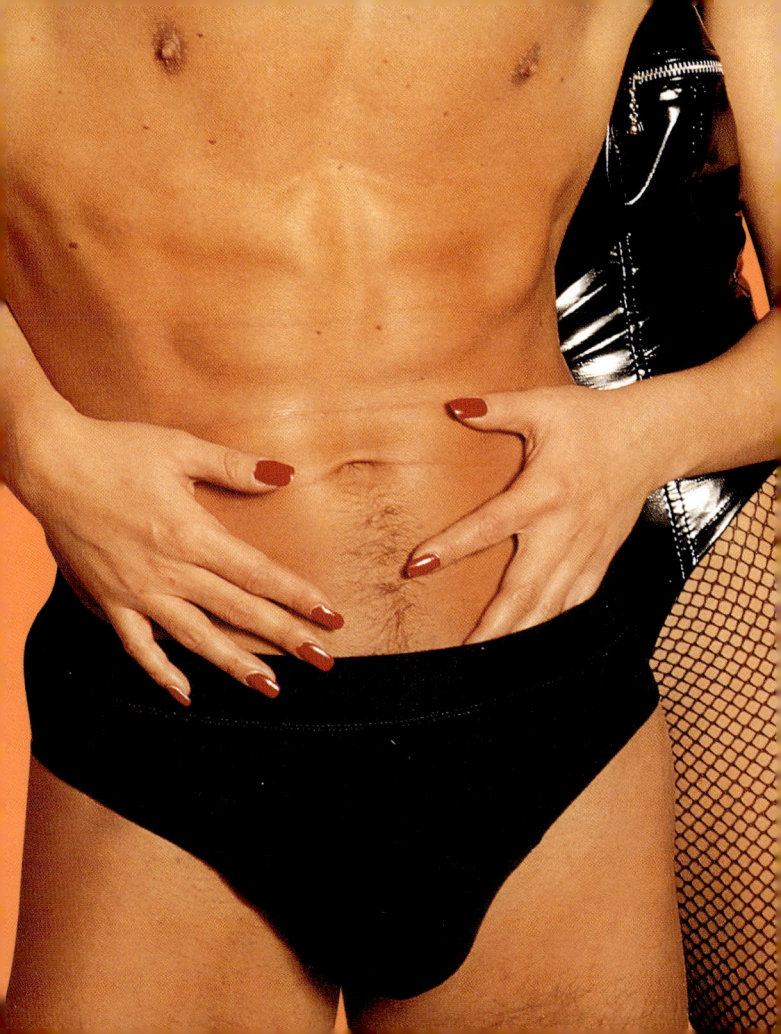

CHAPTER 2
IN THE

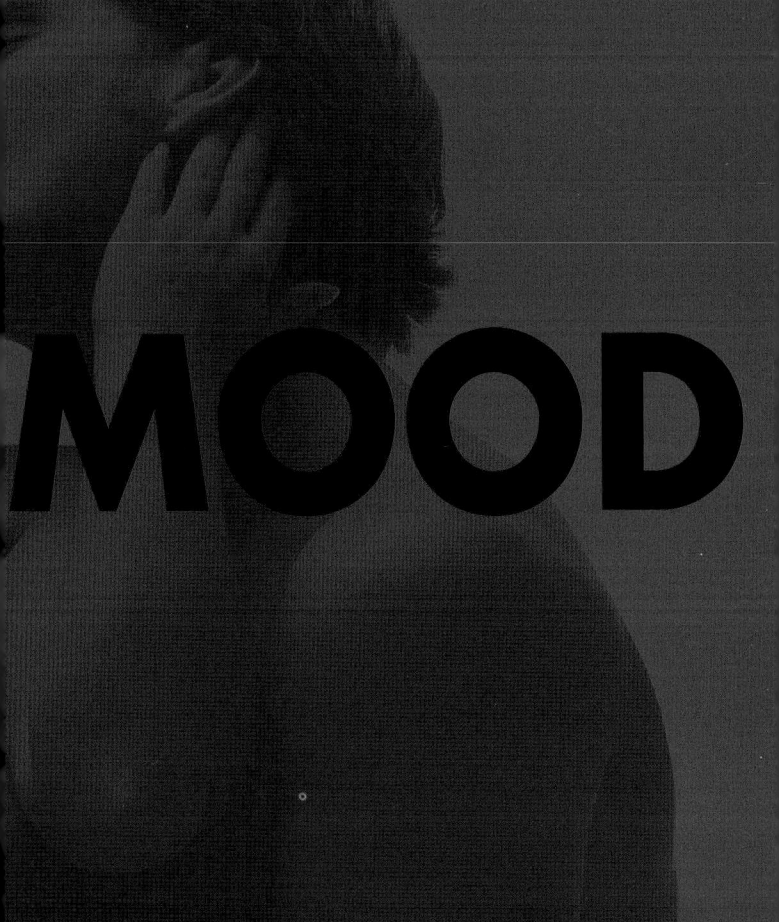

IN THE MOOD

LET'S
KISS

❤ A kiss on the mouth combines the senses of touch, taste, and smell. Start by kissing gently with your lips. Cup your lover's face in your hands and then press more firmly as you part your lips and slowly begin to caress your lover's mouth with your tongue.

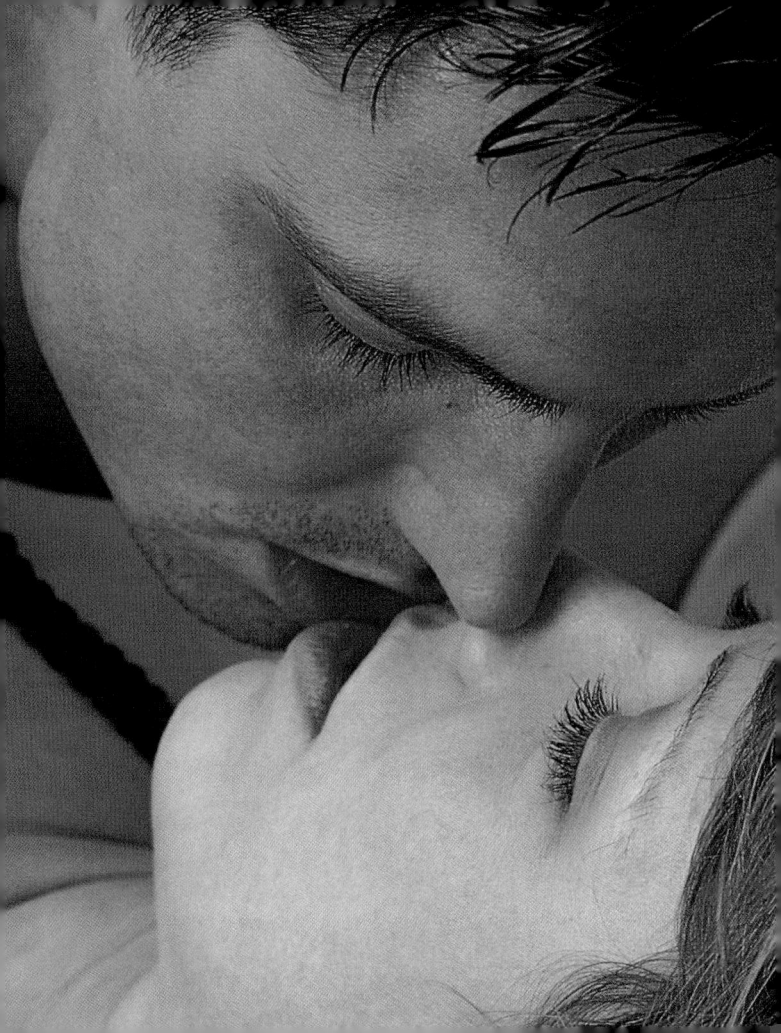

IN THE MOOD

DO-IT-YOURSELF
SEX

❤ Masturbate alone before you see your partner – but don't let yourself reach orgasm. This way you'll be dying for sex when you meet.

❤ Masturbate in front of each other. The first person to reach orgasm has to give the other a sexual favor.

IN THE MOOD

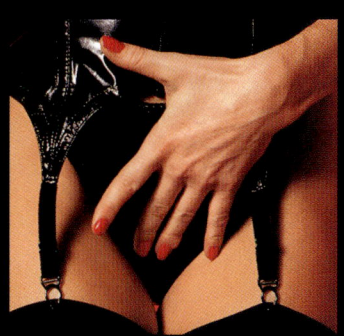

❤ Titillate your partner by masturbating in front of him. Close your eyes and pretend that you're truly alone.

❤ Buy her a masturbation toy such as a vibrator, and tell her that it's solely for her pleasure. Get her to use it on herself as a warm-up prior to your arrival.

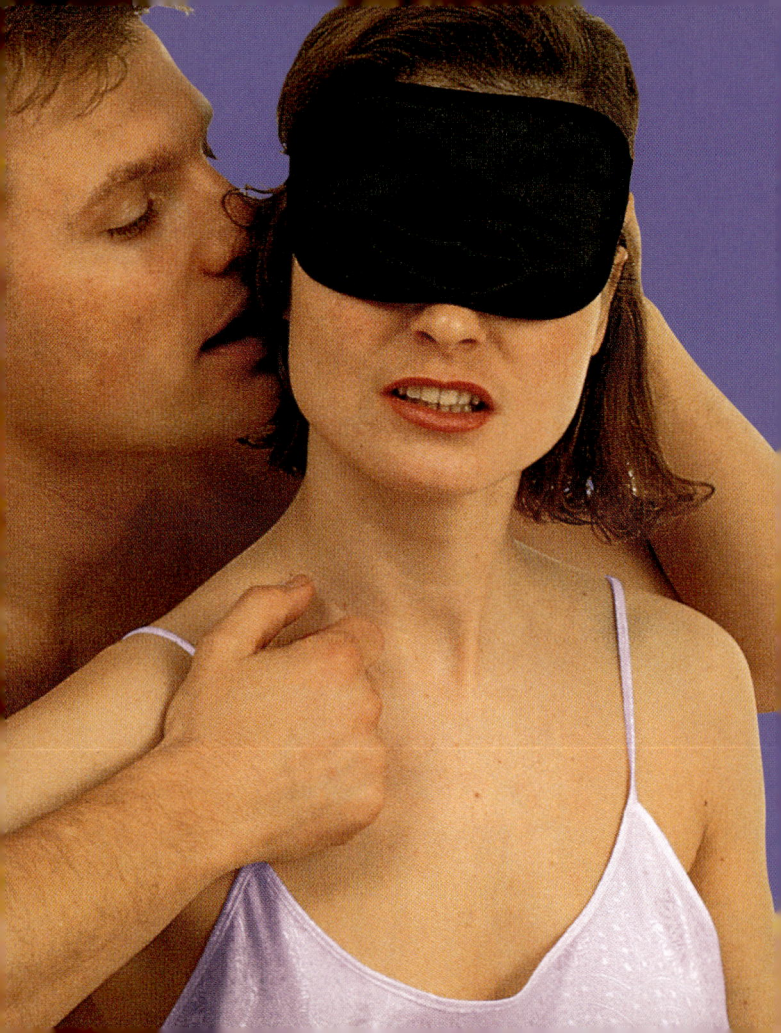

IN THE MOOD

SEX
TALK

❤ Keep her in a state of tingling anticipation by blindfolding her and whispering in her ear what you are going to do to her in bed.

❤ Pay your partner breathless compliments during foreplay. Tell him how sexy he is and how turned on you feel.

❤ Tell sexy stories or anecdotes in bed.

IN THE MOOD

TONGUES AND TOES

❤ Kiss the soles of the feet and draw your fingers between each toe.

❤ Wow your lover's mind by washing her feet in the bath and then sucking lingeringly on each toe in turn.

❤ Pamper him with a peppermint foot bath and rub. Finish by wrapping his feet in a warm fluffy towel.

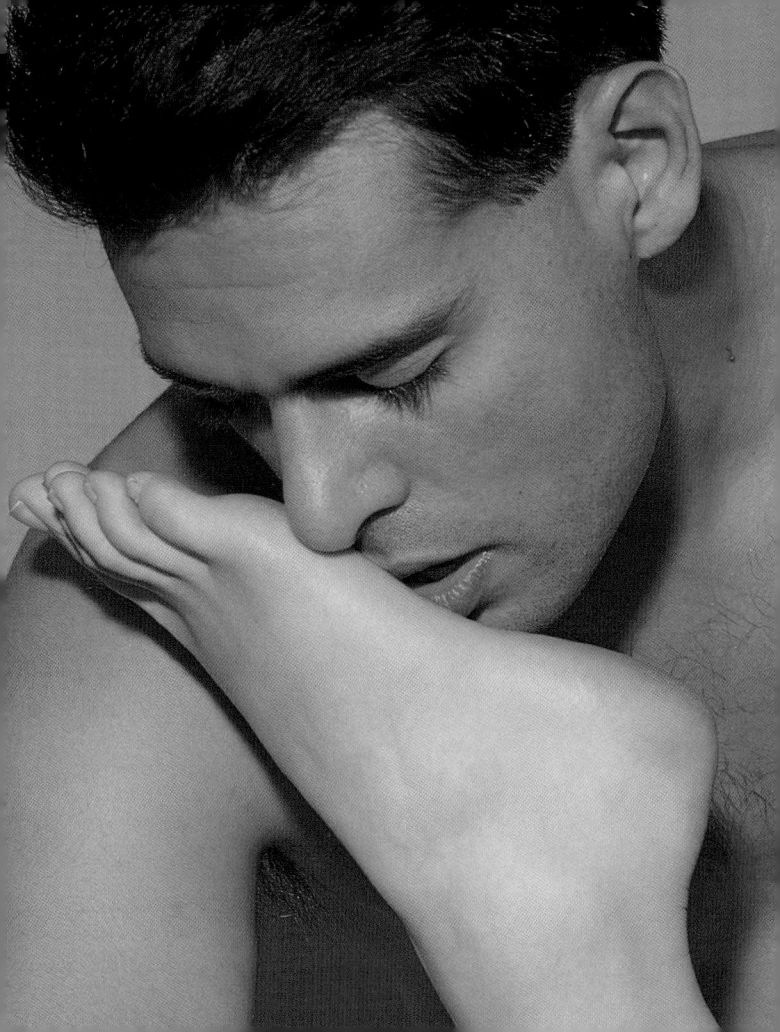

IN THE MOOD

BOUDOIR
BLISS

❤ Make your bedroom into a sexy haven – lots of candles for seductive lighting, a mountain of soft cushions and pillows to fall back upon, and plenty of soft sensual fabrics such as silk, satin, or cashmere.

❤ Scent the air with exotic incense or the fragrance of fresh flowers.

❤ Sprinkle red rose petals on your sheets.

IN THE MOOD

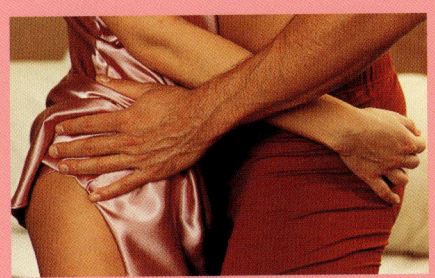

♥ Get rid of telephones, computers, alarm clocks, radios, and anything else that makes a distracting noise.

♥ Put red drapes over your bed or across the window — red is the color of energy and passion.

♥ Keep everything you need, such as massage oils and condoms, right by the bed.

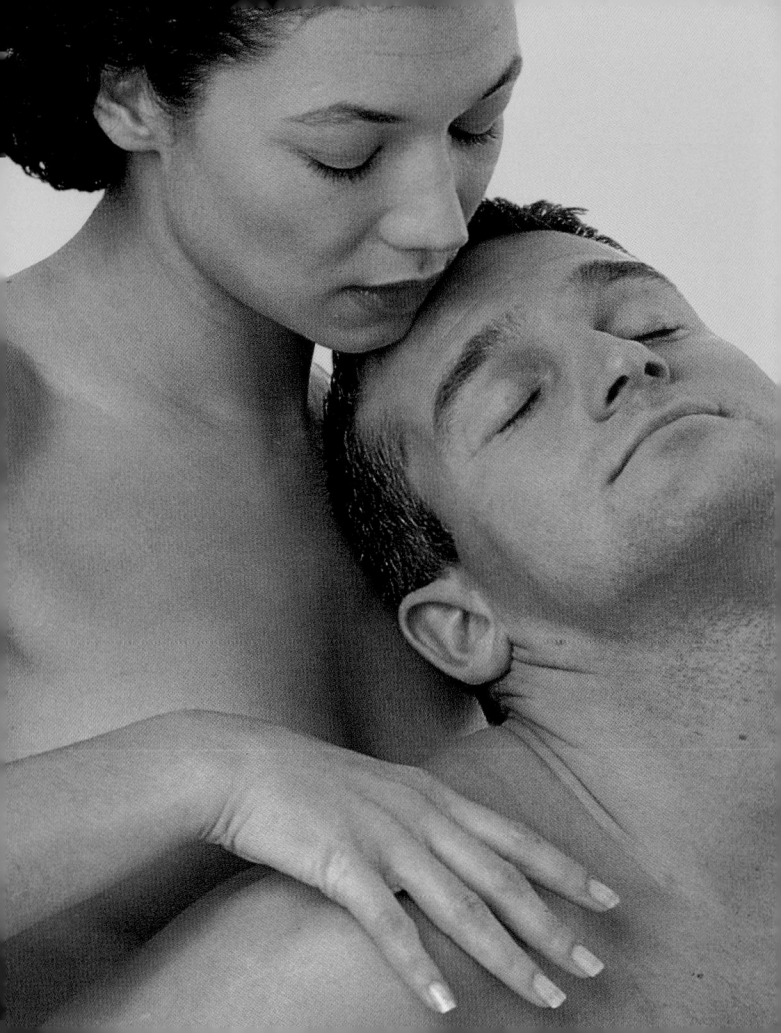

IN THE MOOD

HANDS
ONLY

❤ Give your partner a sensual glow by massaging his neck and shoulders. Rub warm massage oil into your hands and move your thumbs in small firm circles. Afterward, run your fingertips down his back, over his buttocks, and then bring your hands around his front to caress his genitals.

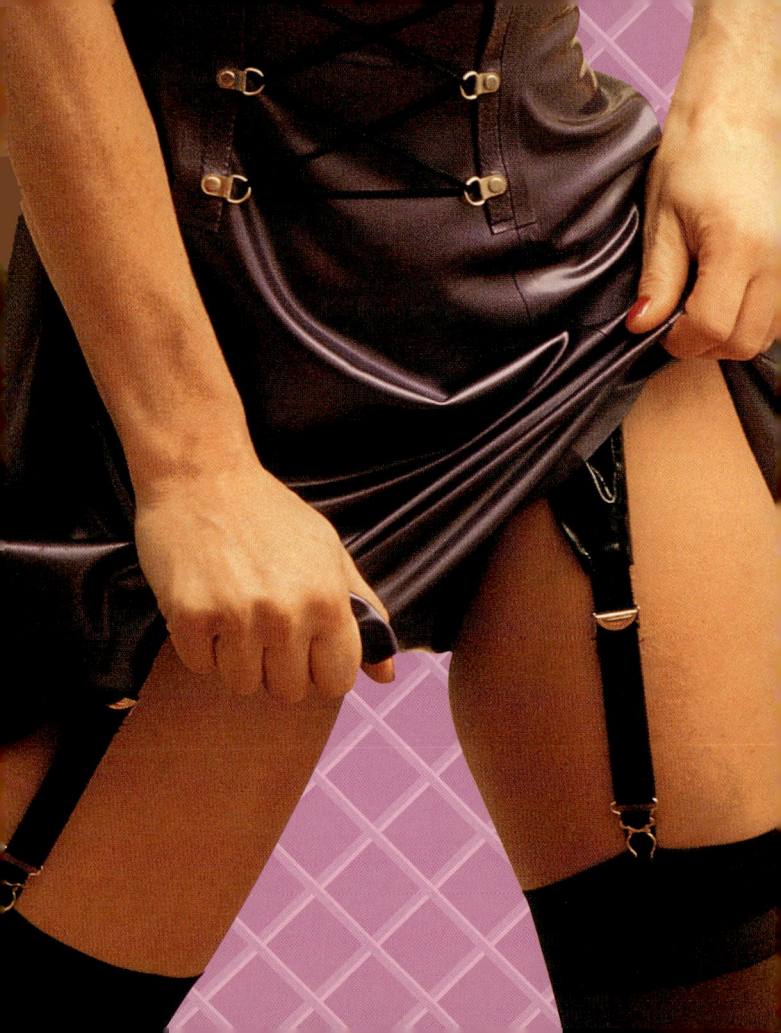

IN THE MOOD

NAUGHTY
NYLONS

♥ Invite him to watch you undress when you are wearing sexy black stockings and a garter. Place one foot on a chair and slowly unroll the stocking down the length of your leg. Drop it on the floor and do the same with the other leg. Let yourself get really turned on by the experience.

♥ Take your stockings off as sexily as possible and then use them to bind your partner's wrists together.

IN THE MOOD

CHAMPAGNE
SEX

❤ Have truly extravagant sex by dowsing each other in champagne and then licking it off. Pour it in each other's navel, and then lap it up with your tongue.

❤ Take a mouthful of chilled champagne and drizzle it over your lover's genitals before you give delicious oral sex.

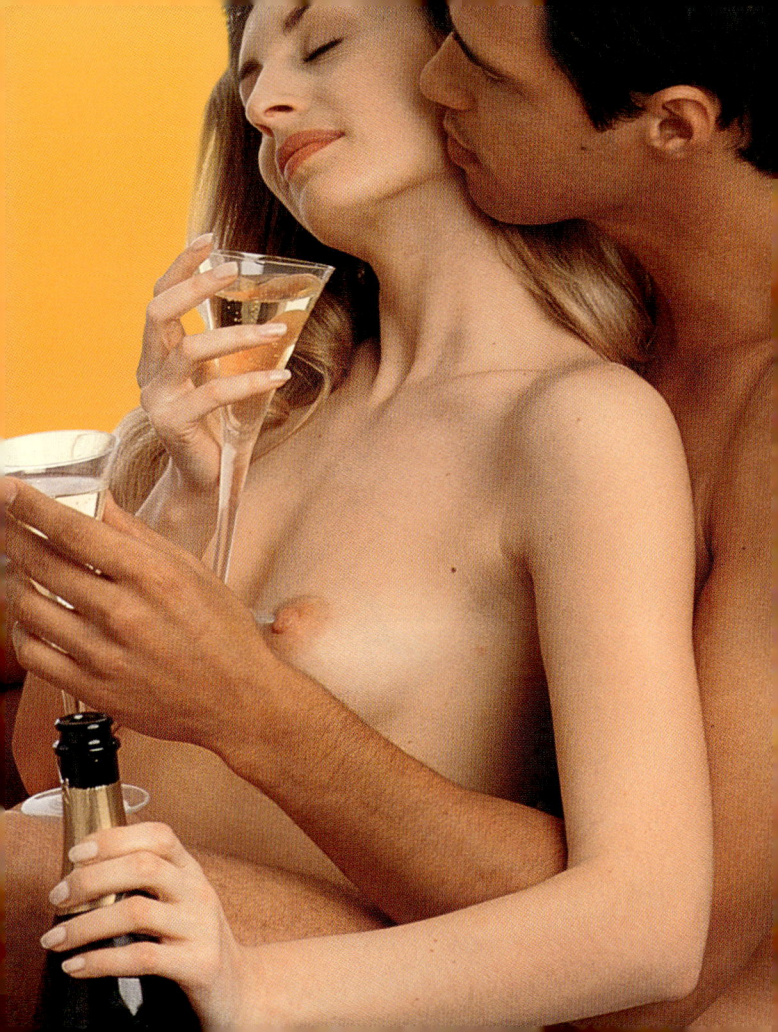

IN THE MOOD

EROGENOUS
ZONES

❤ Wait until she's feeling really aroused and then nibble and nuzzle her earlobe and breathe gently into her ear.

❤ Run your fingertips or nails lightly over his buttocks and trail them down the backs of his thighs.

❤ Pour massage oil on her breasts and then use the head of your penis to massage her nipples.

IN THE MOOD

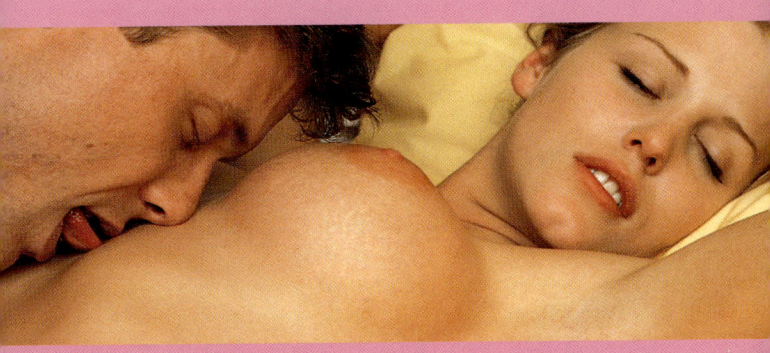

❤ Kiss and stroke him in different places all over his body. Ask him to rate his sensations from 1–5 (5 is amazing).

❤ Spend time kissing and stroking her inner thighs. Don't touch her clitoris – yet!

❤ Use your hair to tickle his belly.

IN THE MOOD

BEDTIME BATH

❤ Treat your bathroom to a romantic renovation. Scatter rose petals in the bath water and fill the room with scented candles. Play some romantic music in the background and share a glass of wine with your lover.

❤ Use a natural sponge to drizzle water over each other's erogenous zones.

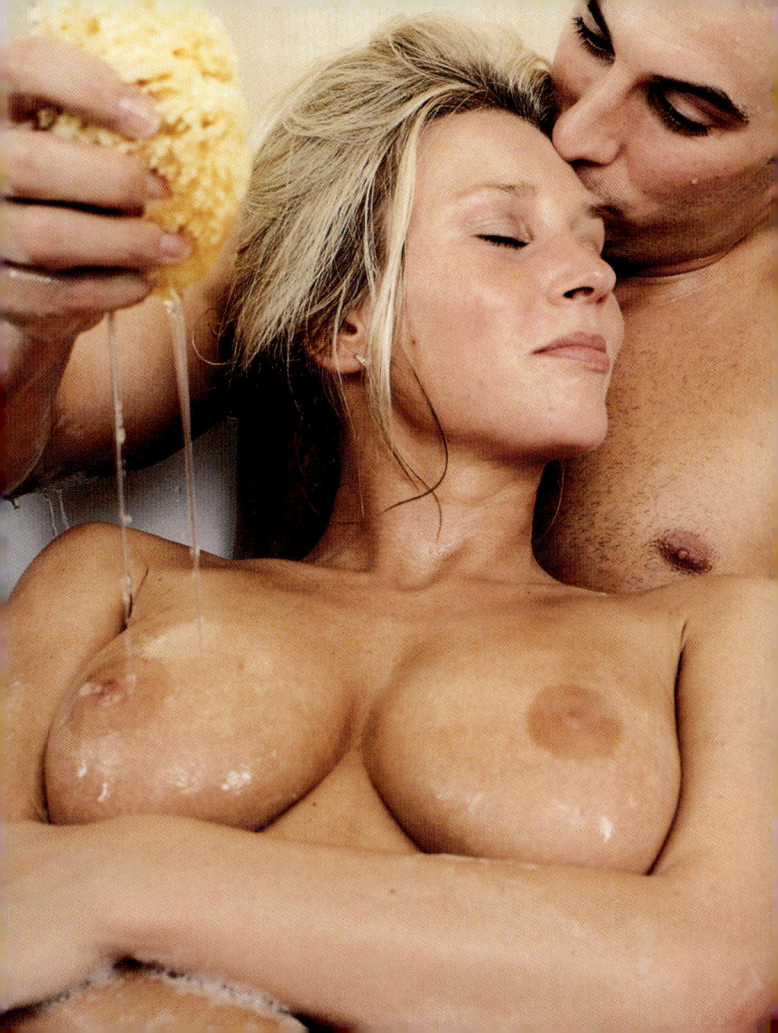

IN THE MOOD

❤ If you're feeling tired ... soak in a hot bath for 10 minutes and then stand up and have a quick cold shower. The pores all over your body will be tingling, and you'll feel invigorated and ready for even the most athletic sex session.

❤ Offer to be your partner's bathtime slave. Your duties include undressing her, soaping her body, shampooing her hair, and, finally, wrapping her up in a big fluffy towel. Then take her by the hand and lead her into the bedroom.

❤ Make bathtime fun by squirting each other with water pistols and playing with rubber ducks.

IN THE MOOD

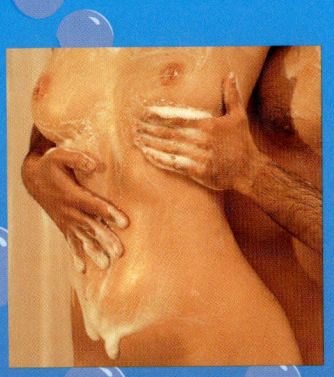

❤ Give each other an orgasm in the bath. Be inventive – use plenty of shower gel, fingers, and toes.

❤ Wash each other's hair, giving each other a glorious head massage in the process – then wash each other's pubic hair, teasing the genitals as you go.

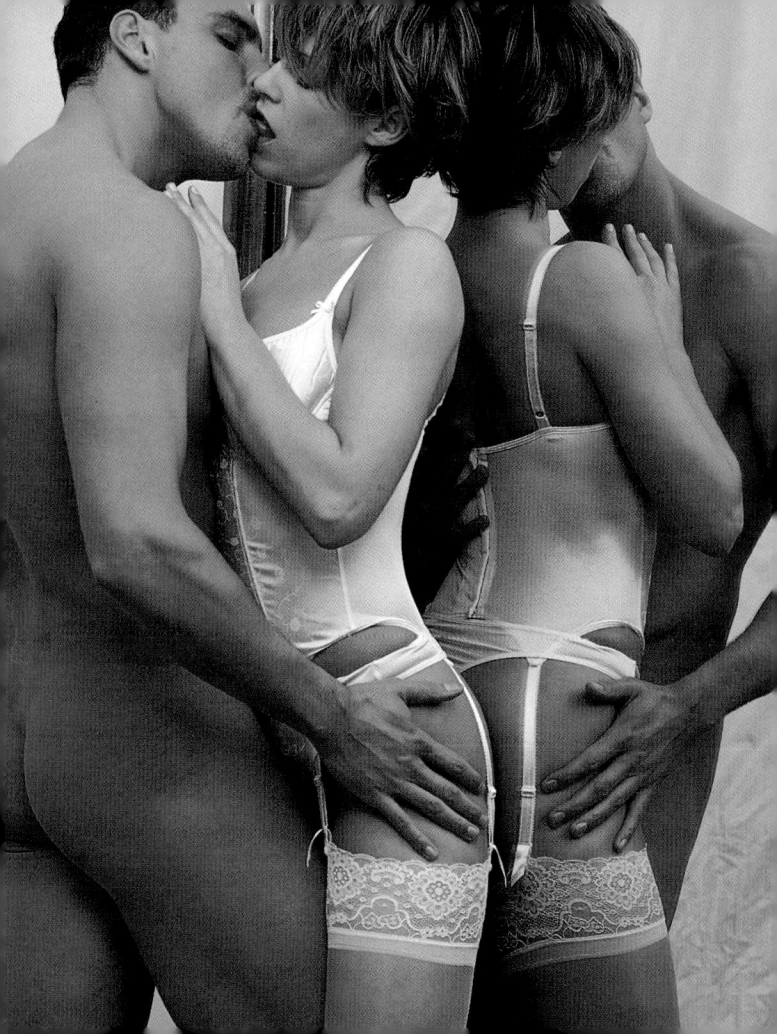

IN THE MOOD

MIRROR
MIRROR

❤ Double the excitement of sex by making love in front of a mirror. Be as raunchy and abandoned as you like.

❤ Turn yourself on solo-style. Caress your body in front of a mirror – pretend that you're performing for a camera. Then bring yourself to orgasm, watching yourself the whole time.

❤ Make love doggie-style with a mirror positioned underneath you on the floor.

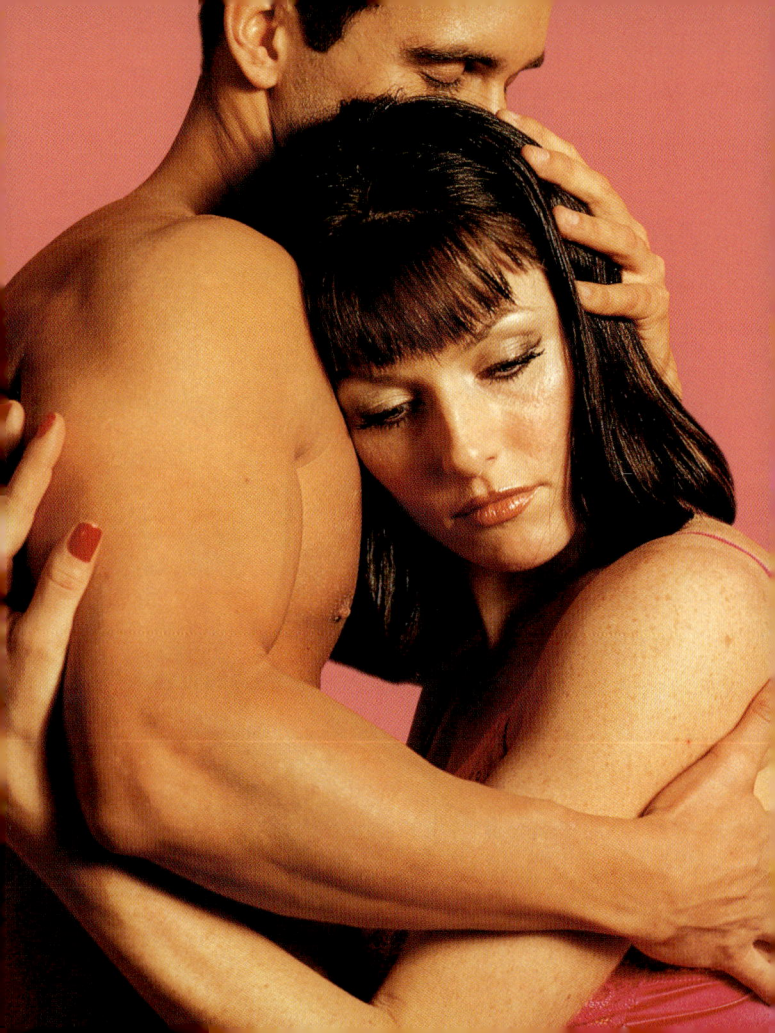

IN THE MOOD

CARESSES AND
HUGS

❤ Spend half an hour caressing before you make love. Don't touch each other's genitals until you've explored the rest of the body first.

❤ Give each other a huge bear hug.

❤ Sneak up behind your partner, wrap your arms around her waist, and nuzzle the back of her neck.

IN THE MOOD

STRIP
TEASE

❤ Start by touching yourself through your clothes.

❤ Take your clothes off extremely slowly and caress your skin as you go.

❤ Look your partner in the eye.

❤ Slip your panties off last.

❤ Enjoy yourself – and show it!

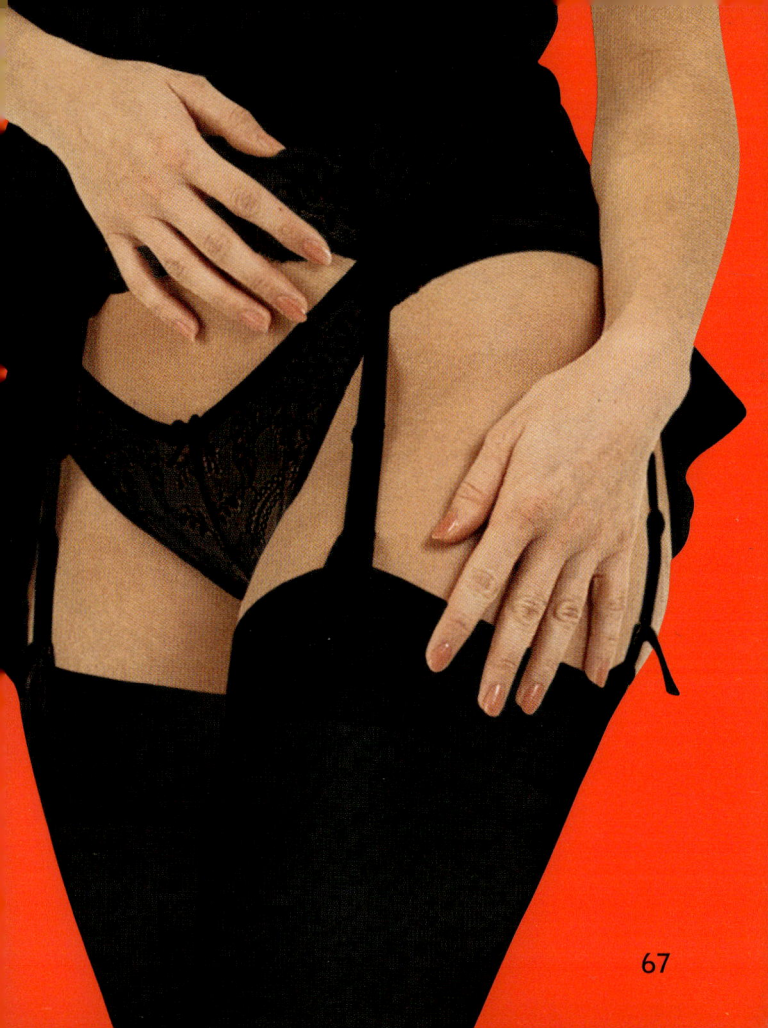

IN THE MOOD

OIL
BATHING

♥ Coat your partner with sweet-smelling massage oil – suntan oil offers a reminder of relaxed days on the beach.

♥ Coat yourself with oil.

♥ Take turns to give each other a long and sensual Indian head massage, using jasmine-scented oil.

♥ Lie down on a big towel and enjoy slippery foreplay together.

IN THE MOOD

❤ Make your hand into the shape of a duck's bill and then drizzle warm oil across the back of your hand so that it drips tantalizingly onto your lover's genitals. Now give a genital massage.

❤ Rub oil into her breasts and nipples.

❤ Beware of using oil and condoms in the same sex session – oil damages rubber and can make condoms ineffective. If you want a slippery lubricant, use water-based jelly or saliva.

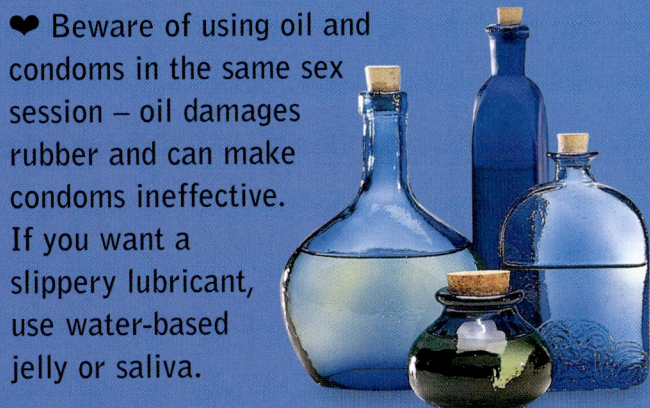

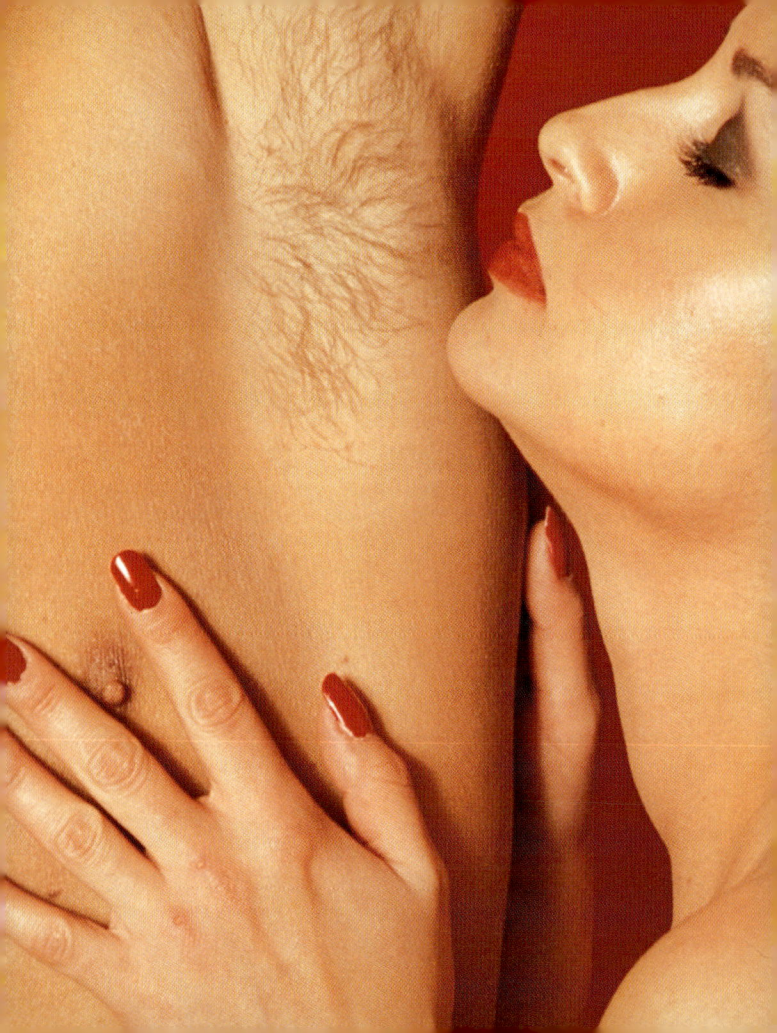

IN THE MOOD

SENSUAL
SMELL

❤ Remember that bodily smells are sexy. Your partner's fresh sweat can be a unique and personal turn-on.

❤ Use exotic Eastern essential oils on your bed sheets and pillows. Try ylang ylang, patchouli, and jasmine.

❤ Spray some of your perfume or aftershave onto a tissue and give it to your partner when the two of you are apart.

IN THE MOOD

WEEKEND
AWAY

❤ Schedule a sexy weekend away a month in advance so you have plenty of time for anticipation.

❤ Don't take anything practical with you. Pack your suitcase with exotic lingerie, sex toys, massage oil, and a saucy present for your partner.

❤ Spend the first evening relaxing with a fantastic sexual massage.

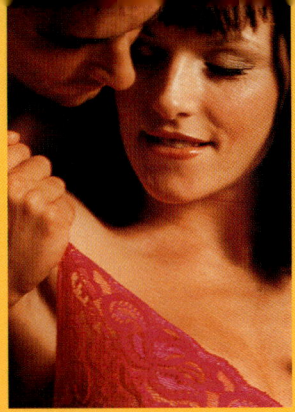

❤ Order some champagne from room service and share a steamy bath together.

❤ Sleep until you wake up naturally, and then spend long lazy mornings in bed teasing and fondling each other.

❤ Make the evenings special. Dress up, share an exotic cocktail in the bar, and choose a restaurant together.

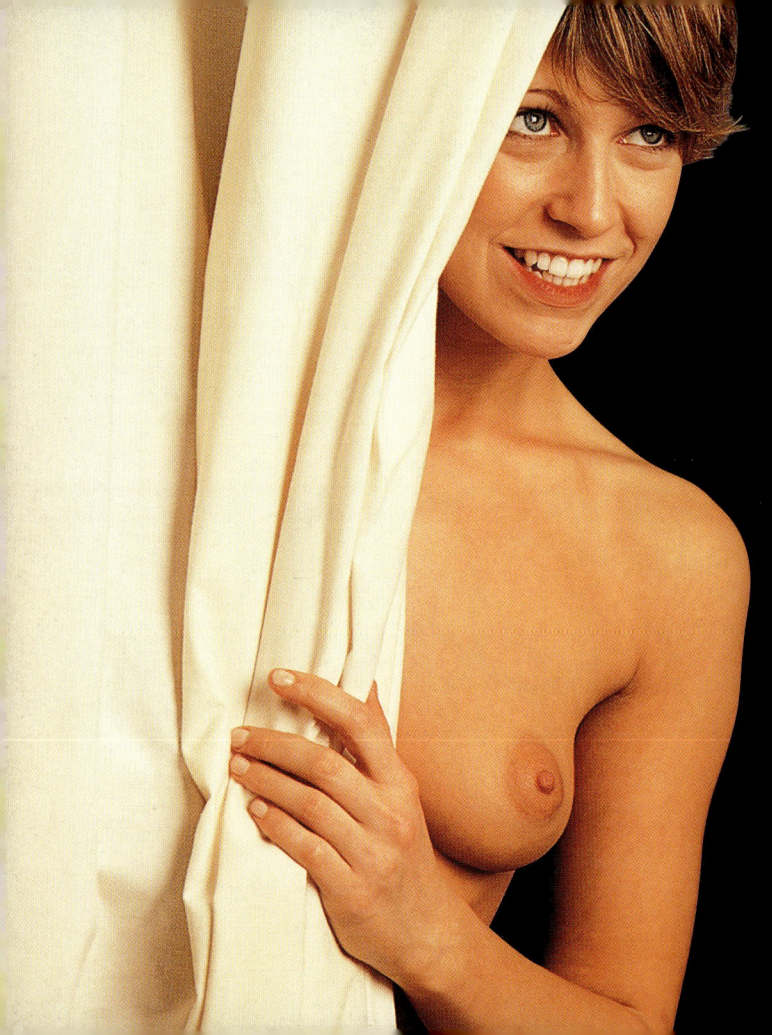

IN THE MOOD

PEEK-A-BOO

❤ Tantalize your partner by draping yourself with a sheet and then letting it slip to "accidentally" reveal a momentary glance of your naked body.

❤ Sexual shyness can be provocative. Keep some underwear on, or cover your breasts or your genitals with your hands. This way your partner feels privileged when you finally reveal all.

IN THE MOOD

STEAMY
SAUNA

❤ Watch your partner's temperature rise as you share a sauna together – even if you can't make love, you can let the sexual tension mount, and then rush home afterward.

❤ Find an excuse to get close by massaging coconut oil into each other's skin and hair.

❤ Take turns to suck on the same mint.

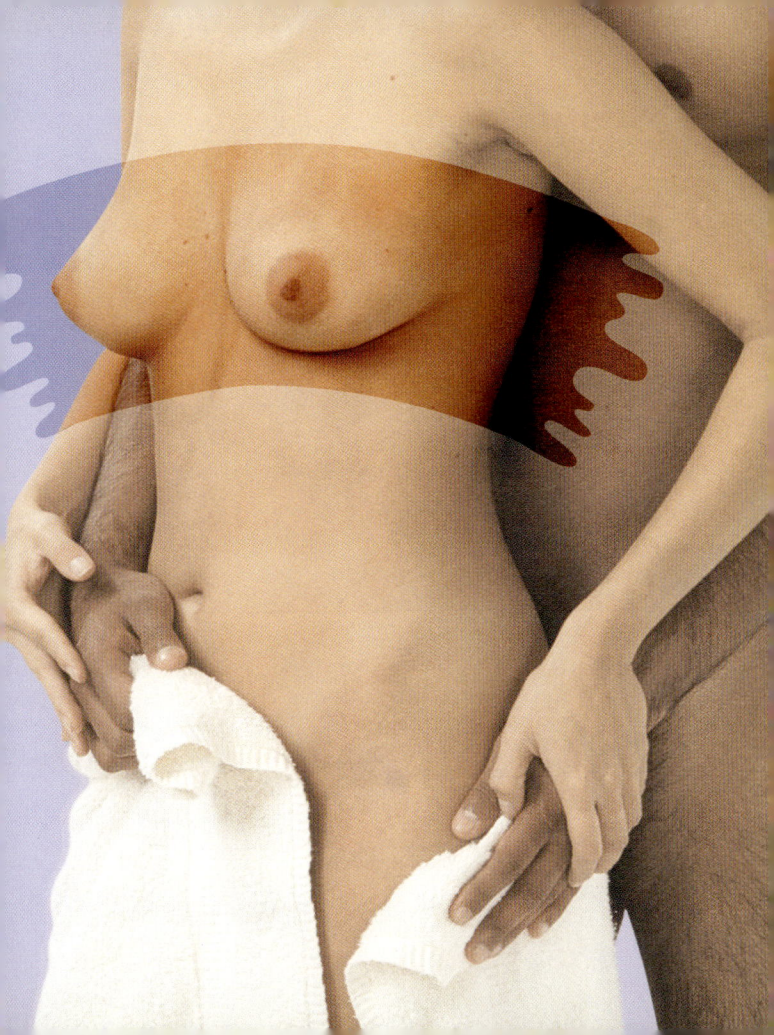

IN THE MOOD

BEDTIME
STORY

❤ Buy a book of erotica and lure your partner to bed early one night with the promise of a special bedtime story.

❤ Print out some erotic stories from the internet. Good websites include www.cleansheets.com and www.eroticaforher.com.

❤ Take turns to reveal your raunchiest sexual fantasies.

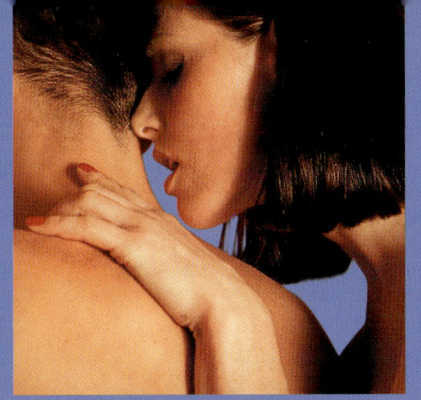

❤ Remind your partner of an exciting and sexy encounter that you've both shared.

❤ Read a sex manual aloud to each other in bed – then follow the instructions.

❤ Write your own erotica and give it to your partner to read alone.

❤ Take turns to create installments of a sexy fantasy.

CHAPTER 3
LOVIN

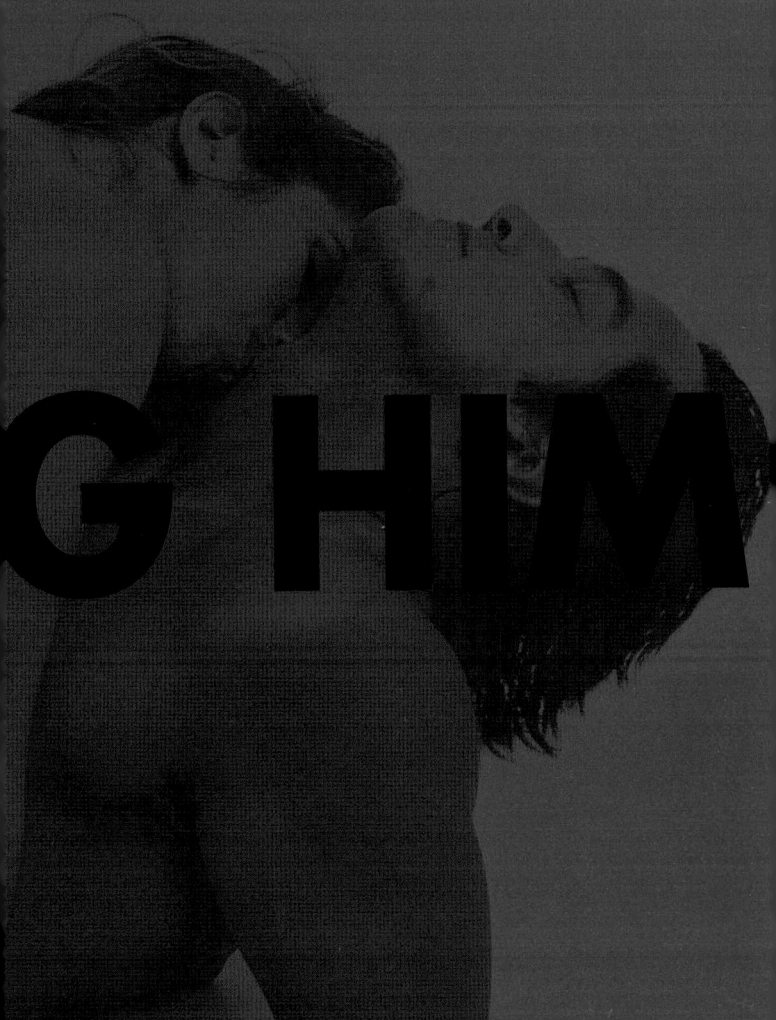

LOVING HIM

BALL
GAMES

❤ Pay special attention to his testicles. Kiss, suck, and nuzzle them. Stroke them underneath at the point where the penis shaft meets the perineum.

LOVING HIM

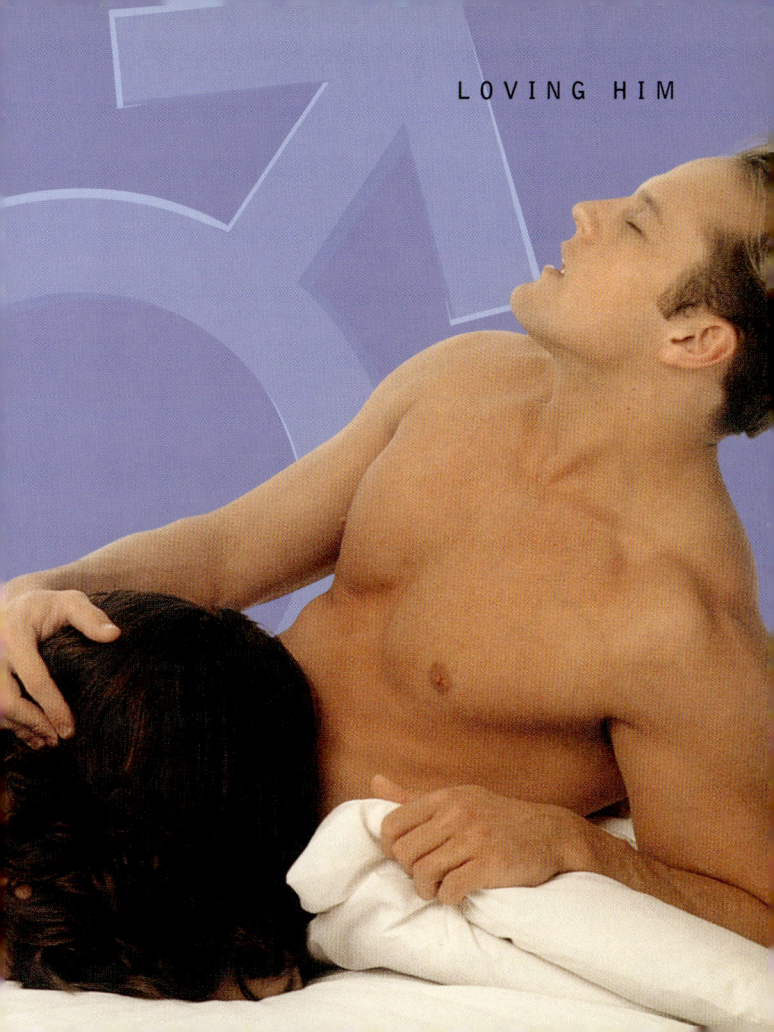

LOVING HIM

PENIS
MOVES

❤ Saliva is a great natural lubricant. Lick his penis all over before you masturbate him – the wetter the better.

❤ Get him to place his hand over yours as you masturbate him. This way he can show you what his favorite speed is and how much pressure he likes.

❤ Caress his penis with unusual textures such as feathers, velvet, or ice.

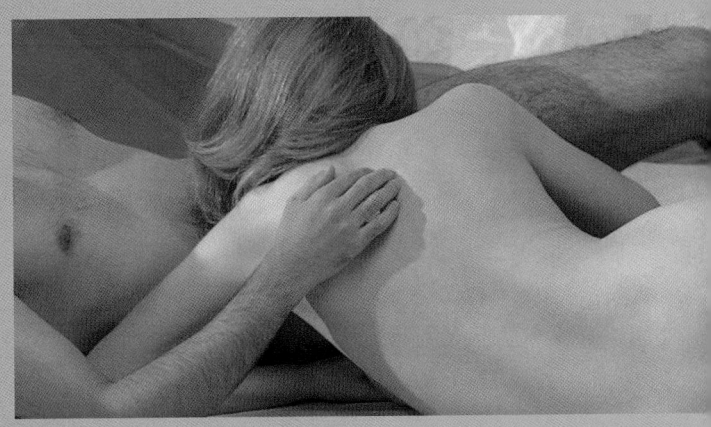

❤ Move one hand firmly up and down on his penis and use the palm of your other hand to rub the head in gentle circles. The contrast between pumping and circling is delicious.

❤ Stimulate his anus with a lubricated finger, as you rub his penis with your other hand.

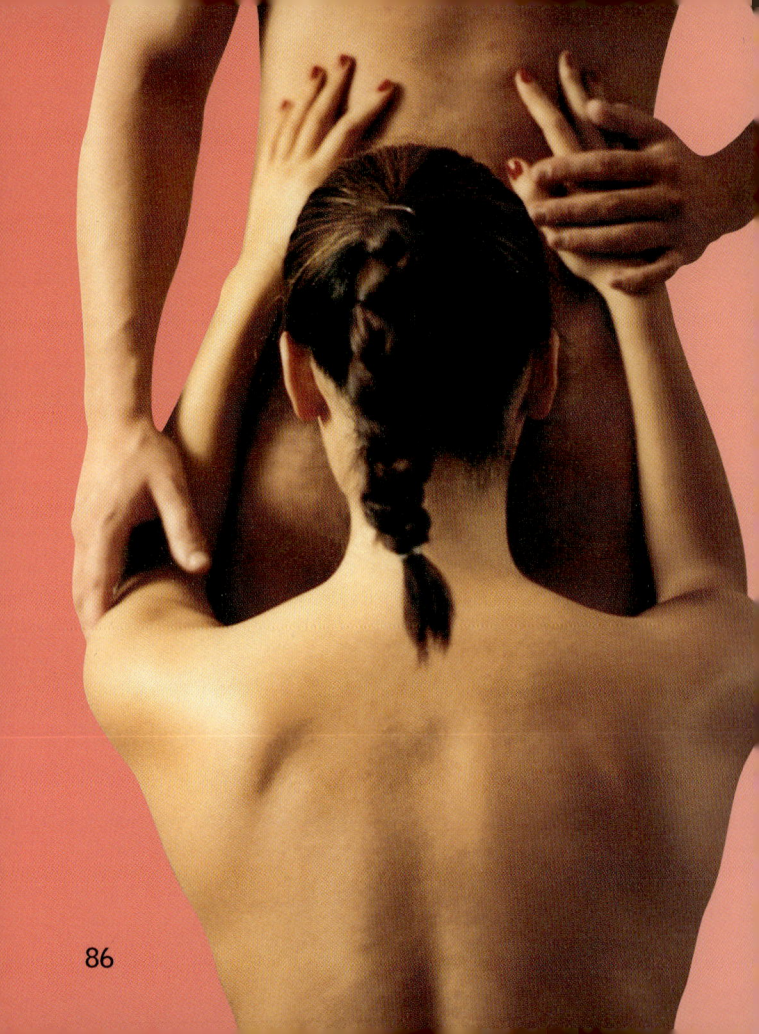

LOVING HIM

ORAL
ECSTASY

❤ Take his penis in your mouth while it's still small. Suck. When he's hard, push your mouth down his penis and set up a pumping rhythm.

❤ Keep him excited by changing the rhythm, pressure, and speed. Look him in the eye.

❤ Hold the base of his penis in your hand, then let him take control by thrusting gently in and out of your mouth.

LOVING HIM

HIP TO
LICK

❤ Turn him on by flicking your tongue all over the front of his body, paying special attention to his nipples, navel, and belly.

❤ Tease your partner with a give-and-take approach. Pull his shorts down and lick the area all around his penis. Get close, but keep stopping short of oral sex. Don't give in until he's reached boiling point.

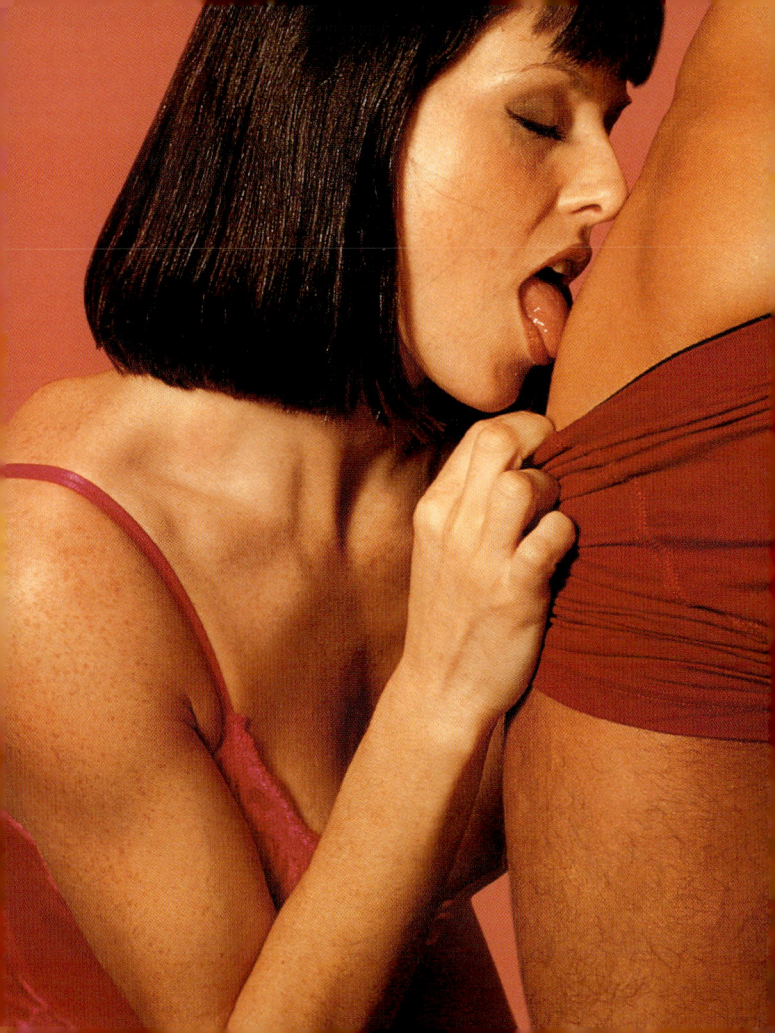

LOVING HIM

THAI **MASSAGE**

❤ This is best done on an inflatable mattress, using a good-quality soap that lathers dramatically. Cover your bodies in soapsuds. Now get him to lie on his back and proceed to "swim" up and down on the front of his body, pushing and wriggling all over him.

❤ Set up a rhythm that stimulates your clitoris – rubbing yourself against his hip or pubic bone, for example. Your pleasure will be infectious!

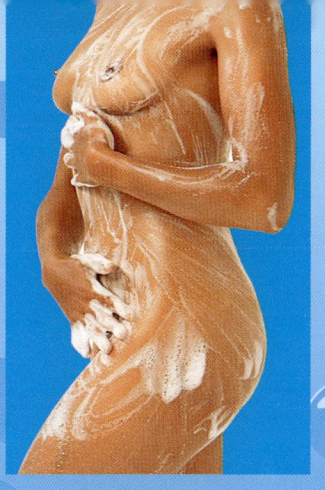

❤ When you slide up and down his front, position yourself so that his erect penis touches your vaginal entrance. As the sexual tempo increases, let his penis penetrate you a little bit. Increase the penetration on each downward stroke.

❤ Keep up the massage until you've both had an orgasm. Then share a hot shower.

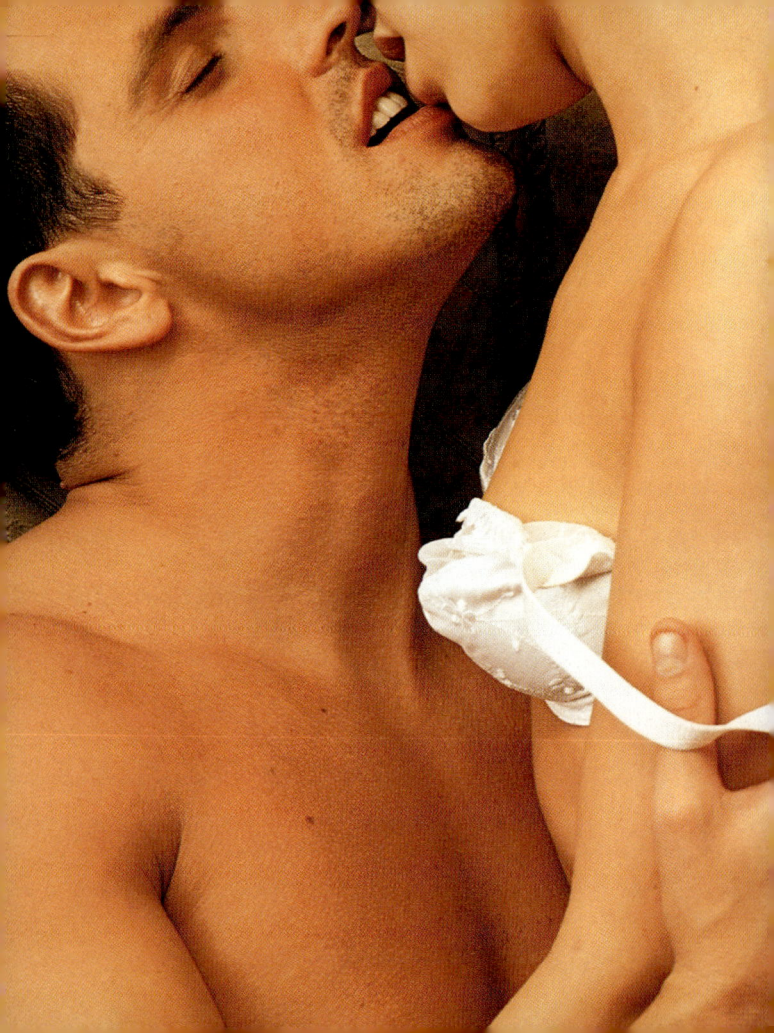

QUICK TRICK

❤ Fast, spontaneous sex is among the best. Forget foreplay and just go with the mood!

❤ A good position for quick sex is standing up. You bend over and he penetrates you from behind – you don't even have to take your clothes off, and you can do it in any room of the house (or office after hours!).

❤ If there's no time for sex, masturbate him while he's fully dressed.

LOVING HIM

PENETRATING POSE

❤ Have sex in positions that allow the penis to deeply penetrate the vagina – this will maximize sensation for your man. Make sure that you're really well lubricated in advance.

❤ Lie on your back and, after your partner has penetrated you, draw your legs up so that your ankles are resting over his shoulders.

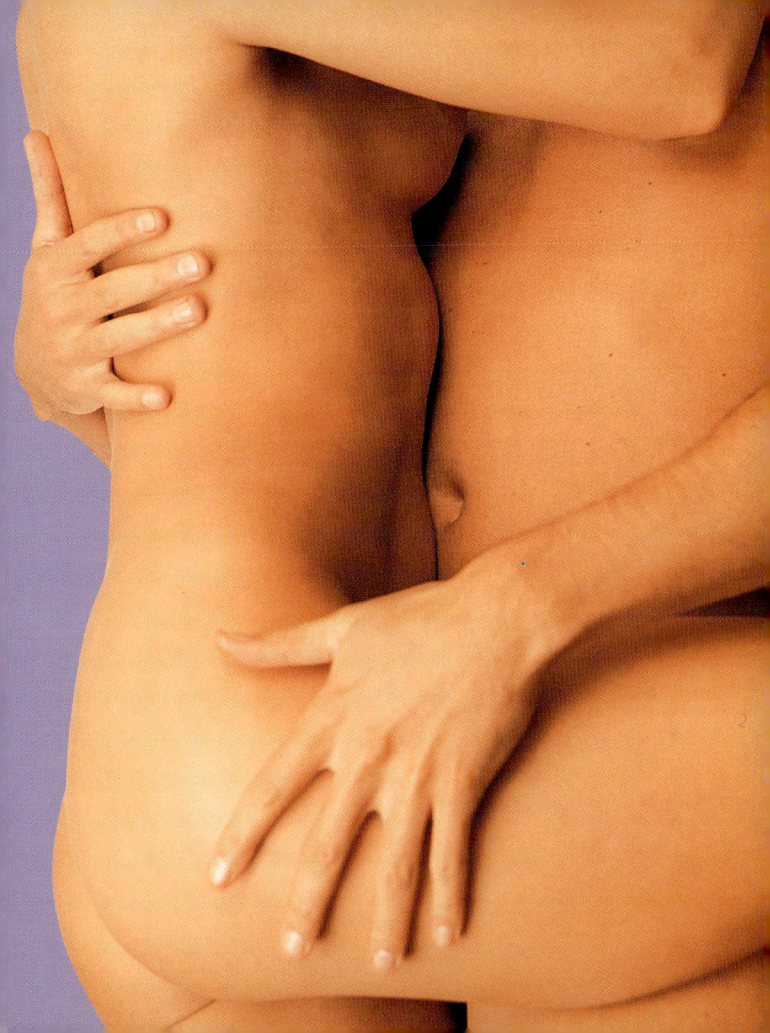

❤ Lean over and put your forearms on the dining room table or have sex on the floor doggie-style – this gives him completely free access to your vagina. You, meanwhile, can stimulate your clitoris by hand.

❤ Let him lie back and relax as you straddle him and let his penis sink deeply inside you. Even if he can't thrust much you can stimulate him by rocking backwards, forwards, and sideways. Lean forward and give him a passionate kiss.

❤ If you've got really strong leg muscles, squat above him when he's on his back. Now raise and lower yourself onto his erect penis. The faster the better.

LOVING HIM

❤ Grab him when he's sitting down. Pull his trousers off and sit astride him with your legs wrapped around his waist. If he's strong and you're light, he can lift you up to have sex in a standing position.

❤ Sit on the sofa with your legs spread wide apart. Invite him to kneel before you.

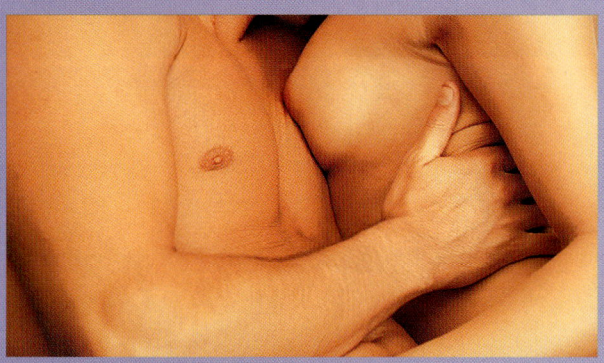

LOVING HIM

THREE-HANDER

❤ Imagine that your vagina is like a third hand that you can use to massage your lover. Make sure that you are both covered in oil, then slip his penis inside you and slide backward and forward while caressing his chest with your hands.
The result: an explosive whole-body experience.

❤ Slip your fingers in his mouth as you make love to him. This echoes the slippery sensation of the penis in the vagina.

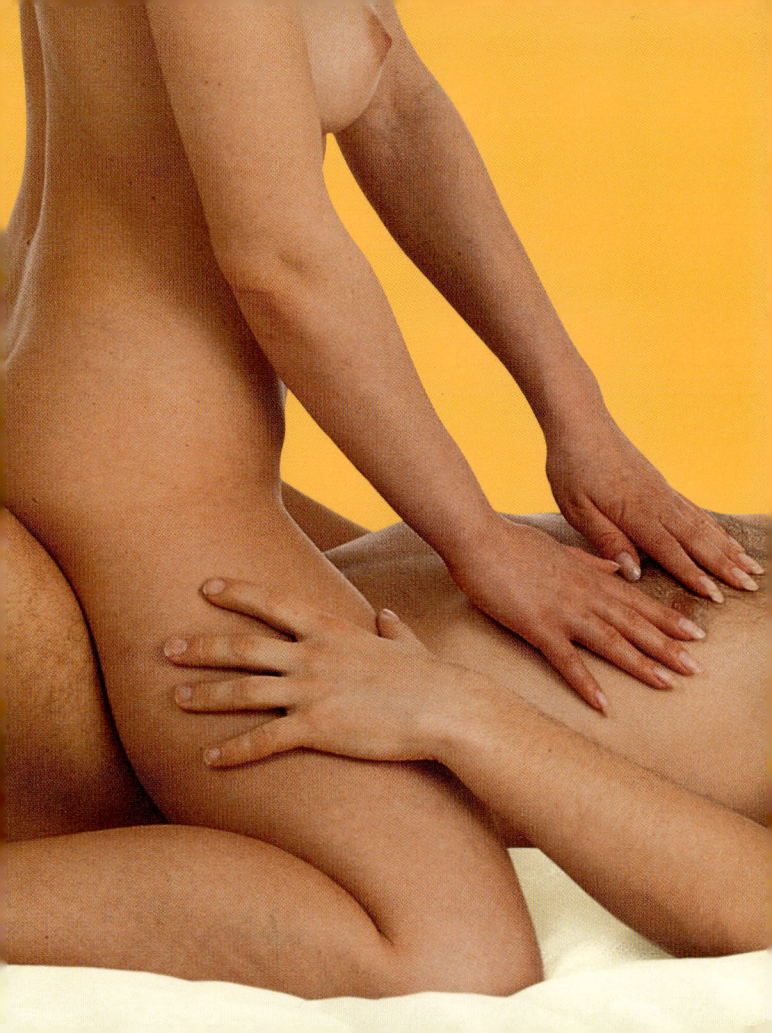

LOVING HIM

VAGINAL
GRIP

❤ Develop a super-fit vagina by squeezing and relaxing your vaginal muscles as if you were trying to stop the flow of urine mid-stream. Now imagine that your vagina is an elevator. Your job is to make it stop and start at floors one to three – both on the way up and on the way down. Practice this every day for the rest of your life! It's a fantastic sexercise – your man will feel like his penis is being hugged during sex.

LOVING HIM

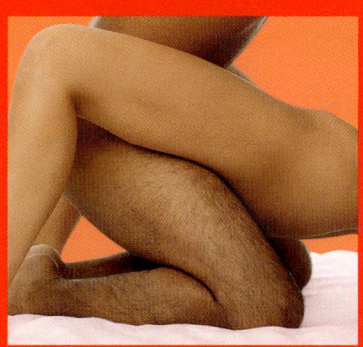

❤ Ask your man to tell you when he's going to climax, and then rhythmically contract your vaginal muscles – this will tip him over into ecstasy.

❤ Have the ultimate in discreet sex – sit on his lap and contract your vagina around his penis while you both stay perfectly still. Close your eyes and concentrate.

LOVING HIM

MEGA-ORGASM

❤ Tell him how horny he makes you feel while he is making love to you.

❤ Grab his buttocks and pull him deeply into you with each thrust when you sense he's about to climax.

❤ Use a vibrator on his anus during sex.

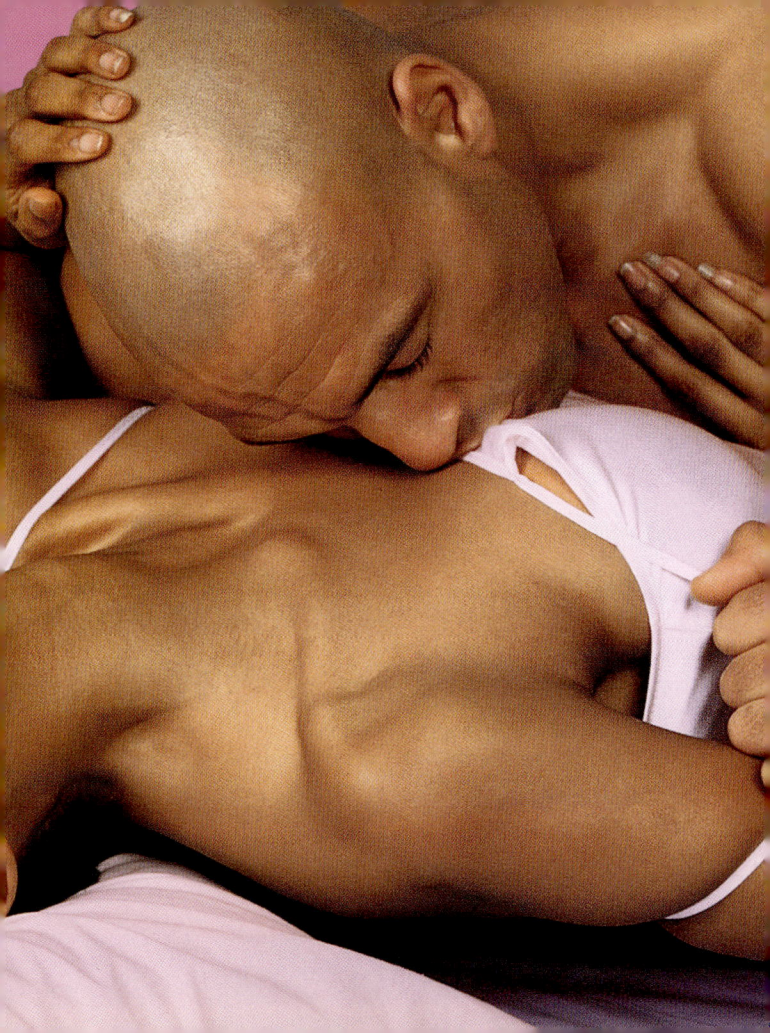

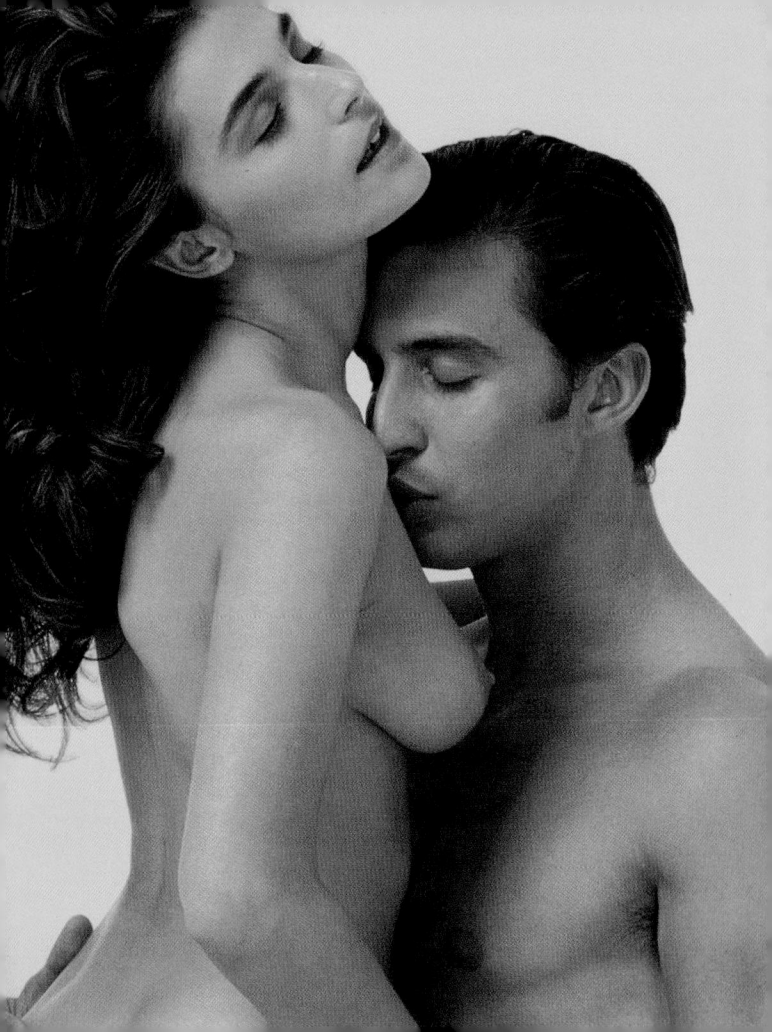

LOVING HIM

PROLONGING THE
PLEASURE

❤ Spend hours on sensual foreplay. Don't touch his genitals until he's desperate to make love to you.

❤ If you think he's about to climax, pull away and take a sex break or turn the erotic intensity down a notch. Spend some time stroking each other.

❤ Teach him the art of yogic sex. Deep breathing and muscle relaxation will help him to delay ejaculation.

LOVING HIM

SPIT AND
POLISH

❤ Fasten your lips firmly over your teeth and slowly engulf your man's penis, sliding your mouth down as far as you can comfortably go. Cover him with your saliva. Move your lips back up his shaft and wrap one hand firmly around the lower part of his penis. Now move your hand and mouth in a synchronized pumping movement. Alternatively, you can vary the sensation by pulling your mouth and hands in opposite directions!

LOVING HIM

❤ Prepare to stimulate him by giving the palm of your hand a long and sensual lick with your tongue and then wrapping it around the shaft of his penis.

❤ Alternate hand stimulation with oral sex. Not only will you keep him guessing, but you'll never run out of lubricant, and your mouth won't get tired!

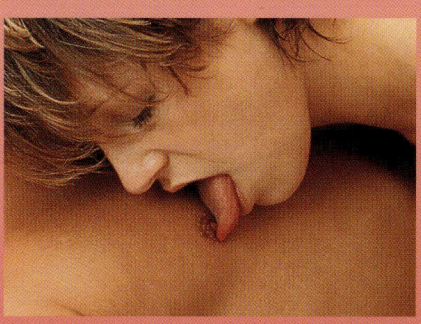

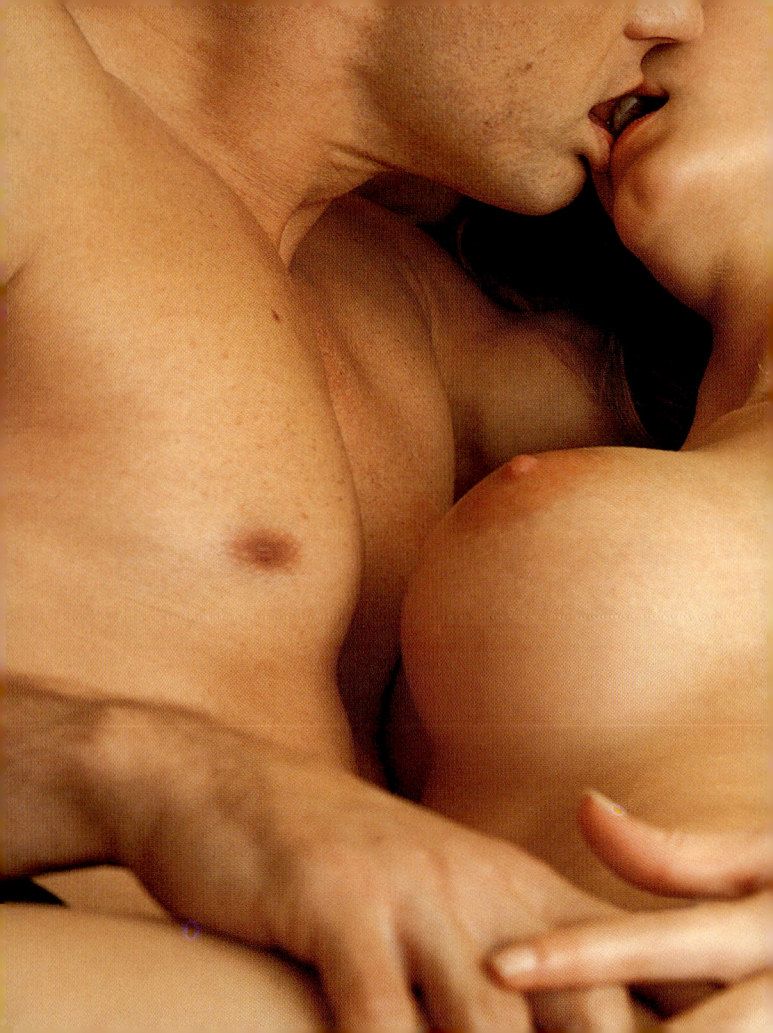

MORNING CALL

❤ As your lover lies innocently asleep, whisper in his ear "this is your wake-up call, darling." Gently stroke his body under the sheets, and brush your hand over his penis. Kiss his face until he wakes up.

❤ For a hard-core wake-up call, massage his penis until it's erect and then make love to him. Or put his penis into your mouth. Check that he'll like this in advance though!

LOVING HIM

CLEAVAGE
CARESS

❤ Wear a push-up bra or outfit that emphasizes your cleavage, then lean forward and invite him to give you a breast massage.

❤ Massage your breasts with oil (in front of him for maximum titillation), then lie on top of him and use your breasts to lubricate the front of his body.

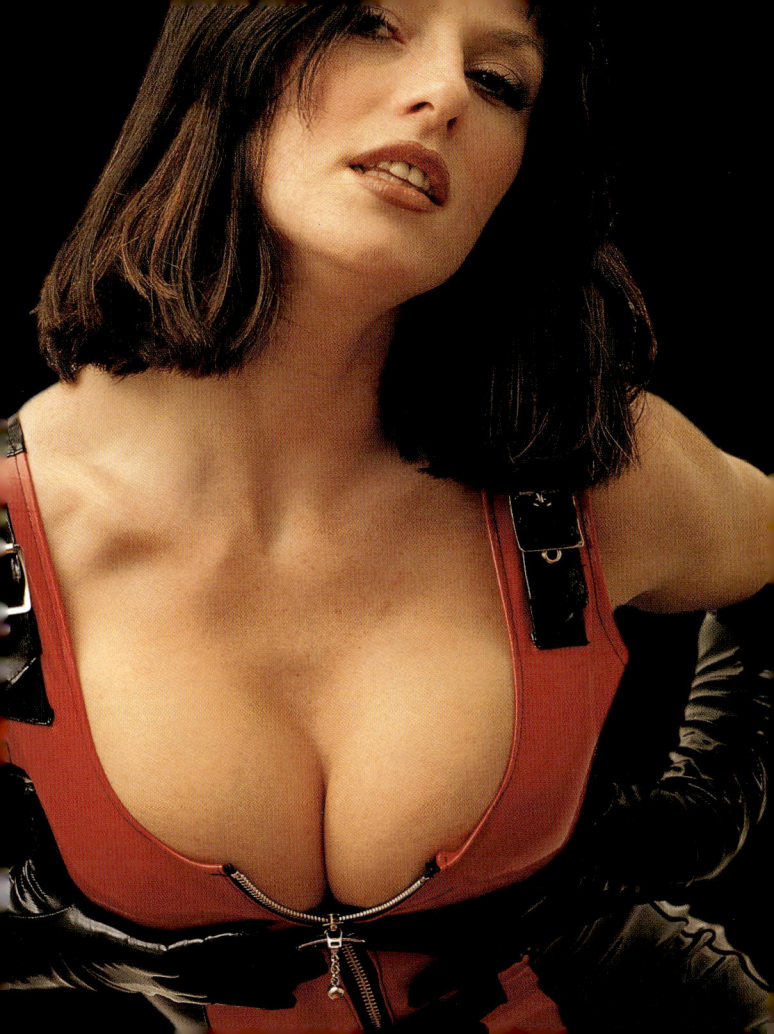

LOVING HIM

CONDOM
TRICKS

❤ Practice your skills on a cucumber, so that you can apply a condom to a penis in seconds flat.

❤ Keep condoms under your pillow to reduce fumbling time.

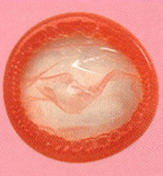 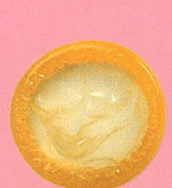 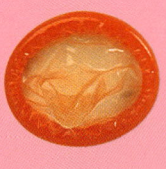

LOVING HIM

❤ Hold the tip of a rolled-up condom between your lips during oral sex. As you slide your mouth down his penis, you can also unroll the condom.

❤ Keep some water-based lubricant nearby.

❤ Give your lover condoms in sexy colors and shapes when he's least expecting them: on a plate instead of dessert, or at a party with a whispered invitation to visit the bathroom, for example.

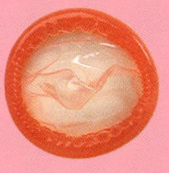
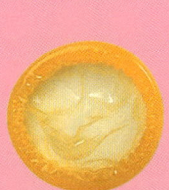
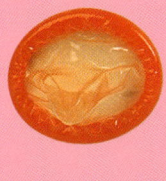

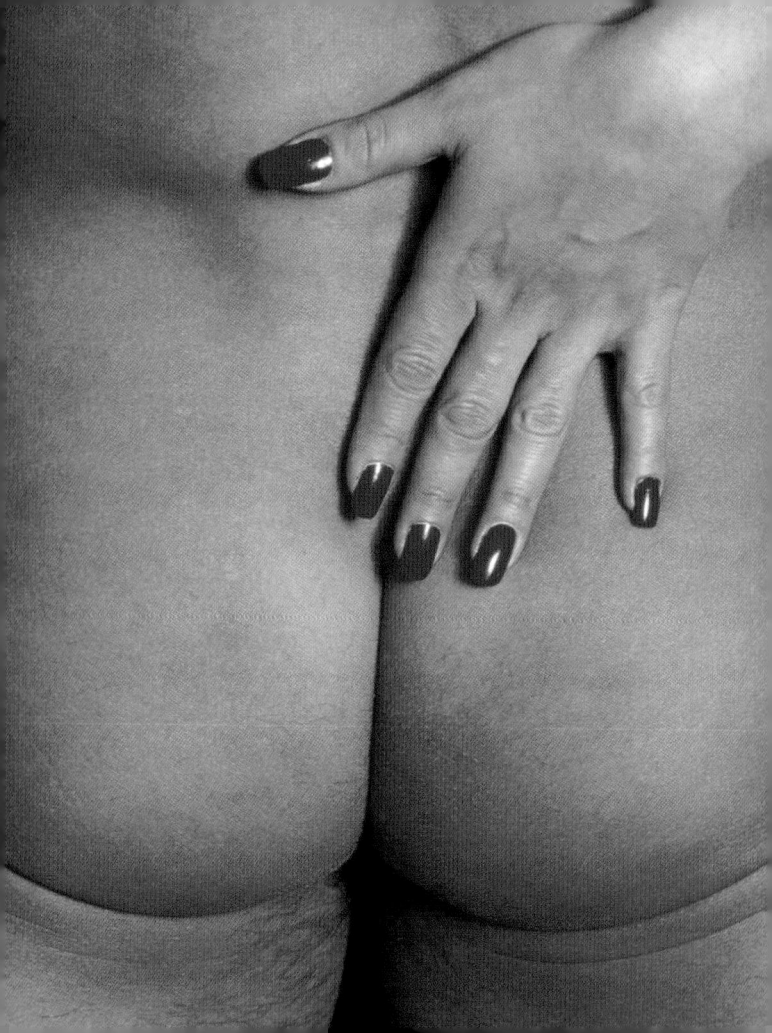

LOVING HIM

HOT
SPOTS

❤ Find your lover's personal hot spots and exploit them to their full erotic potential. Is it his buttocks, his lips, the nape of his neck, his feet, or the insides of his thighs that really get him going? Don't ask – experiment!

❤ Don't forget that men have nipples, too. Find out how sensitive your man's are by licking, flicking, teasing, and caressing them. Try out some nipple clamps on him.

CHAPTER 4
LOVIN

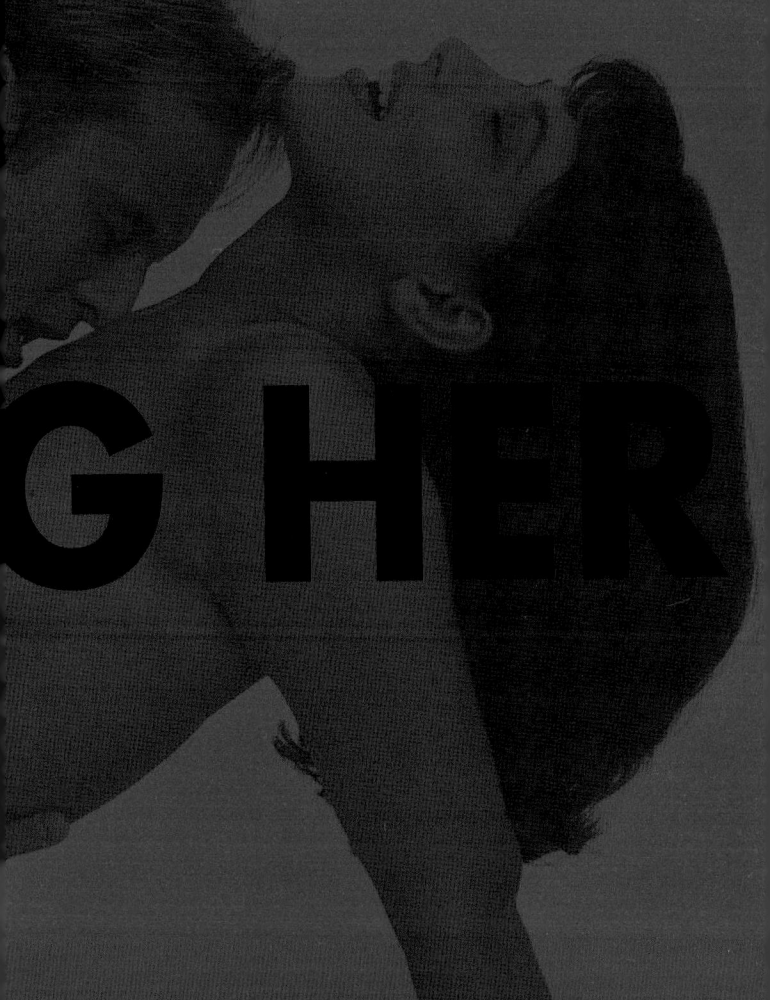

LOVING HER

G-SPOT
MAP

♥ Pressing your lover's G-spot can trigger orgasm. The G-spot is found about two-thirds of the way up on the front vaginal wall.

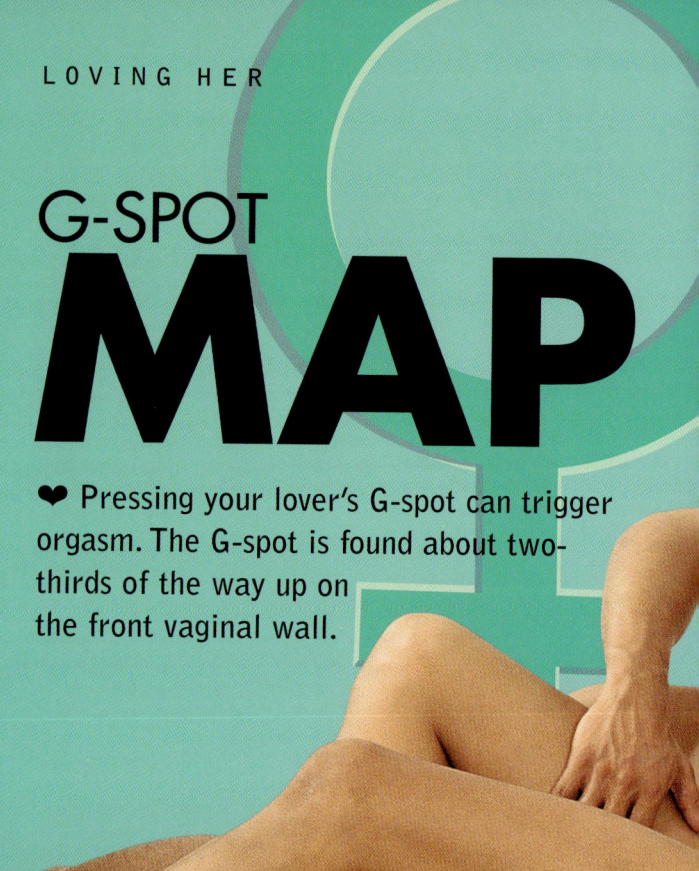

LOVING HER

❤ Try different types of touch and pressure on the G-spot to see what she likes most. Unlike the clitoris, which needs lots of friction, many women prefer a static touch on the G-spot.

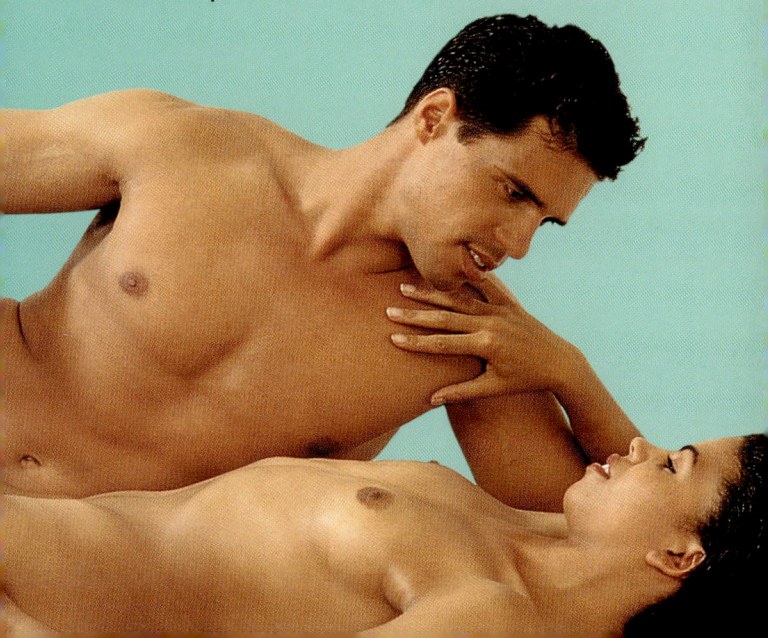

LOVING HER

❤ Play the "hot and cold" game. Explore different parts of her vagina with your finger and get her to rate each touch as hot, cold, or – hopefully – boiling point.

❤ Stimulate your lover's G-spot with your penis by penetrating her from behind so that the penis hits the front vaginal wall.

❤ Buy your partner a vibrator that's specially designed to target the G-spot. Look for one with a tip that's gently curved or angled.

❤ As you stimulate her G-spot from the inside, get her to press down on her belly from the outside.

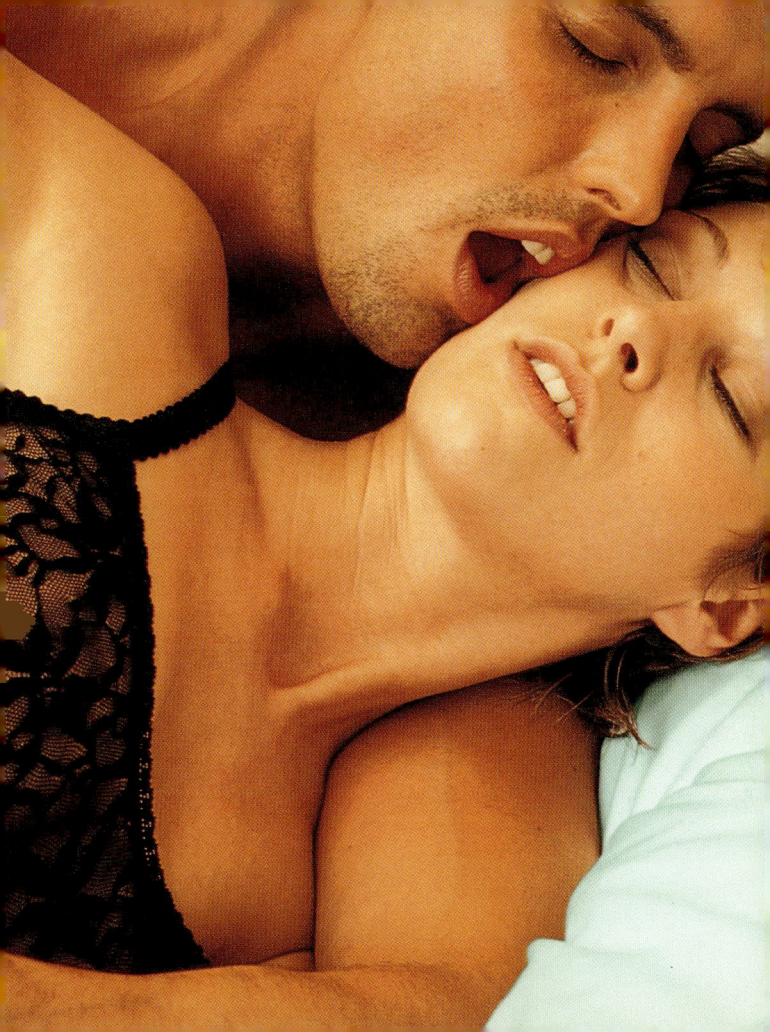

LOVING HER

MASSAGE
BELOW

❤ Never underestimate the sensitivity of your hands and fingers. Eighty two percent of women can climax from masturbation – that's fifty percent more than can climax from intercourse alone.

❤ Use the hand-riding technique. She puts a guiding hand on top of yours while you masturbate her. This way she can show you exactly how fast and how firmly she likes to be touched.

LOVING HER

❤ The clitoris is the erotic hotspot – try rubbing it in circular or backward and forward movements – but don't neglect other parts of her genitals. Try tugging and stroking her labia and massaging the inside of her vagina.

❤ If she's really sensitive, stroke her gently with your fingertip through fabric.

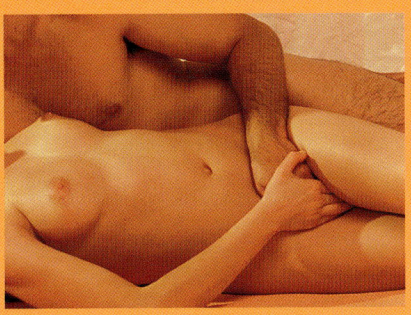

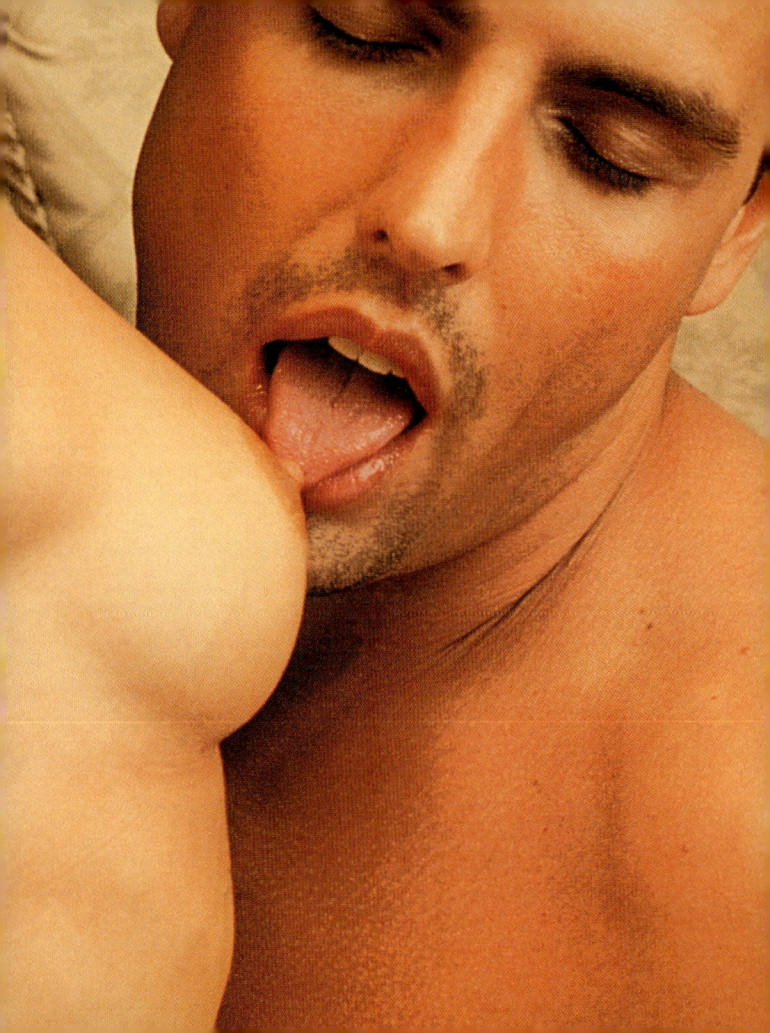

LOVING HER

TONGUE
BATH

❤ Paint your lover with cream or ice-cream and lick her all over. Let her know how delicious she tastes.

❤ Let your lover see your sensual intention. Point your tongue before lapping her body.

❤ Move slowly down her body toward her biggest erogenous zone – the clitoris.

LOVING HER

CLITORIS
STROKES

❤ Position your head between and slightly below her thighs so that you can stroke your tongue upward against the shaft of her clitoris.

❤ Occasionally insert your tongue into her vagina.

❤ Use your tongue in different ways: curl it, flick it, use the blade, and then the tip.

❤ Touch her G-spot as you lick her clitoris.

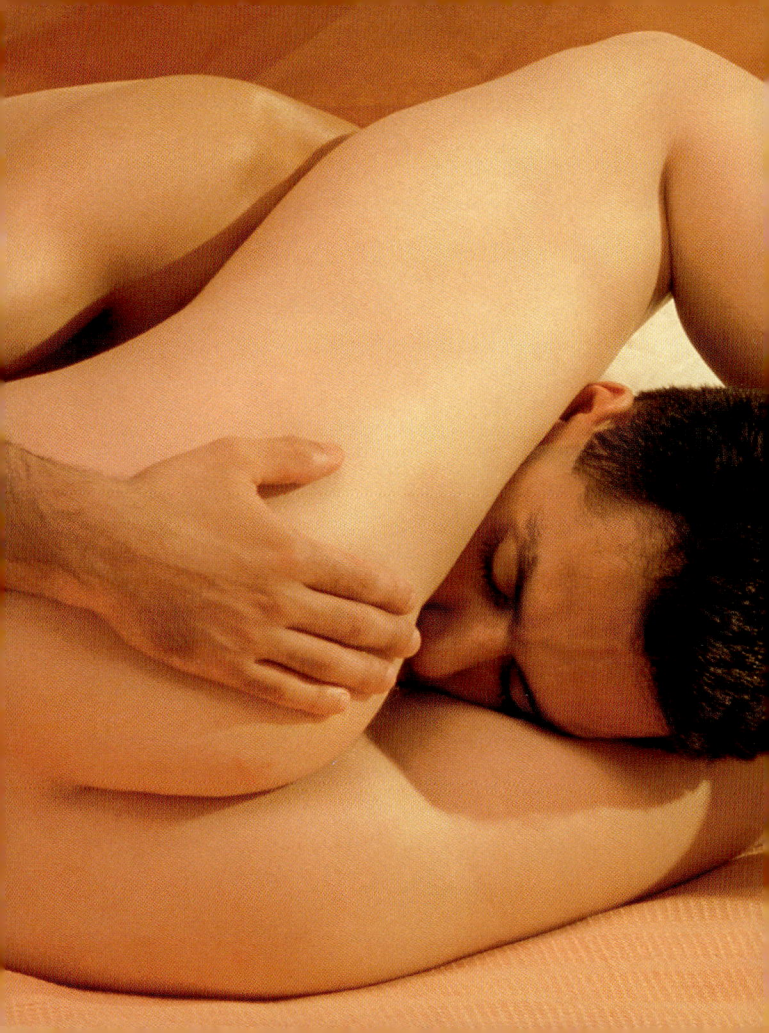

LOVING HER

❤ Once you have tantalized her into total helplessness, try gently covering the clitoris with your mouth and flicking your tongue across it at the same time.

❤ Featherlight tongue-twirling on the top of the clitoris can be fantastic.

❤ If you get tired, let your fingers take over for a while.

❤ Let her direct your head with her hands.

❤ For a really turbo-charged experience, try massaging her vaginal entrance with a vibrator as you caress her clitoris with your tongue.

LOVING HER

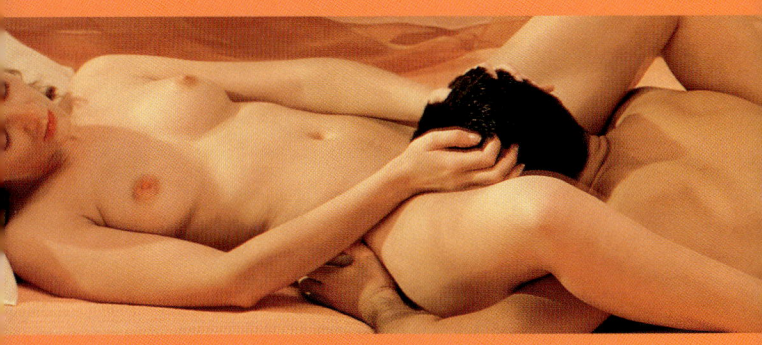

❤ Ask her how she likes it: fast, slow, gentle, rough, hard, soft? If you try something new, ask her if it feels good.

❤ Once you've got into a rhythm that you know she likes, don't stop, slow down, or change the pressure. Keep going until she climaxes.

LOVING HER

TWO
PAIRS

❤ Two pairs of hands are better than one. Next time you make love, get her to caress one part of her body while you caress another part. You can add to the effect by blindfolding her.

❤ Alternatively, if she feels self-conscious, you can wear the blindfold.

❤ While she rubs her clitoris you can give her a sensual G-spot massage.

LOVING HER

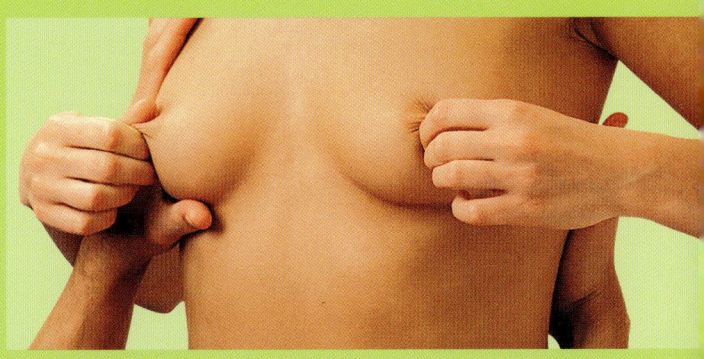

❤ Get her to rub and tweak her nipples while you caress the whole of her breasts.

❤ Stimulate her clitoris until she is close to climaxing, then ask her to rub her belly with her hands.

❤ Add even more sensation by introducing a vibrator to the equation.

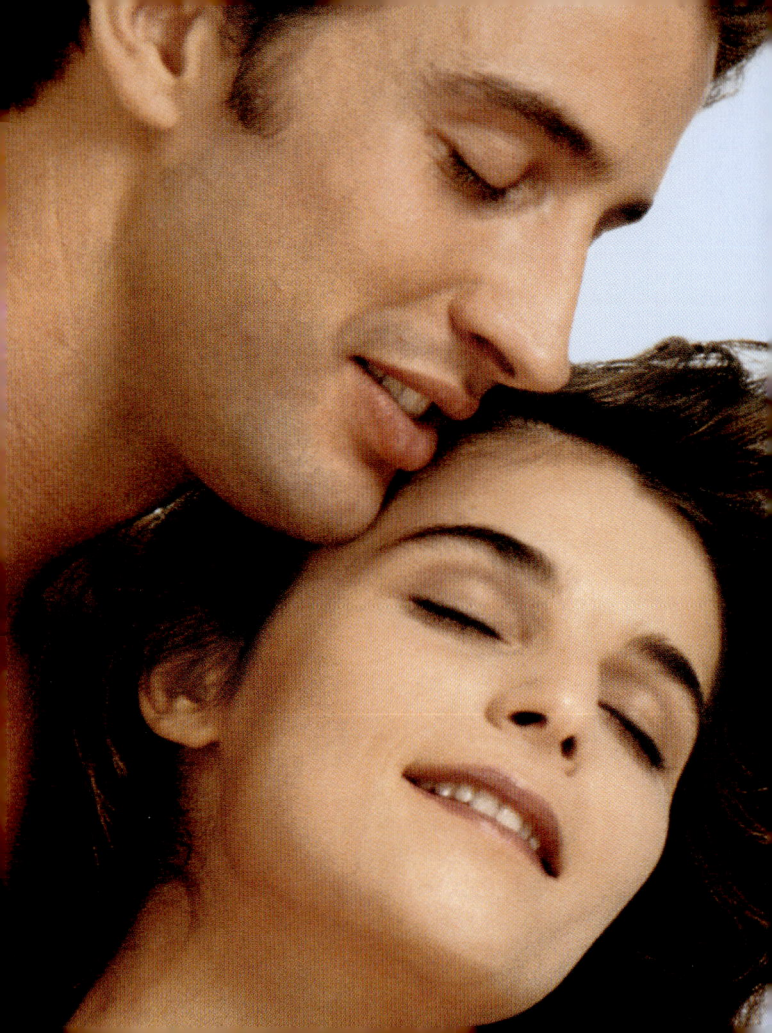

LOVING HER

TENDER
TALK

❤ Say your partner's name as you make love to her.

❤ Tell her how beautiful she is, how much you love her or how much her body turns you on.

❤ When you're out together whisper that you can't wait to get home and make love.

LOVING HER

NIPPLE
TEASERS

♥ Make her nipples tingle with excitement by sucking and then blowing on them. Or, for dramatic erotic effect, lick her nipples with an ice-cube concealed in your mouth.

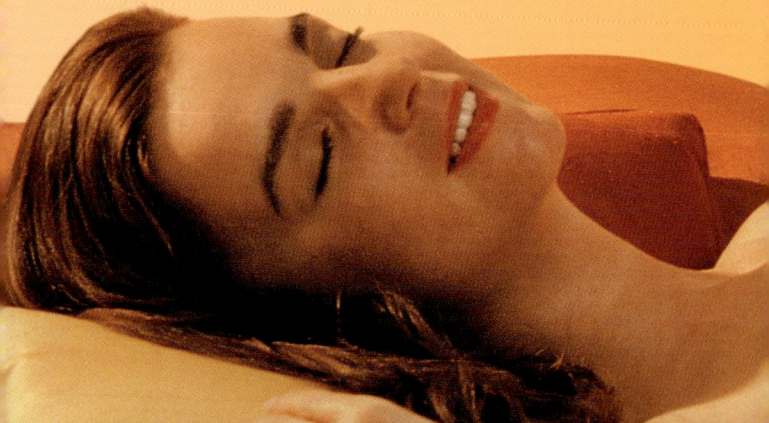

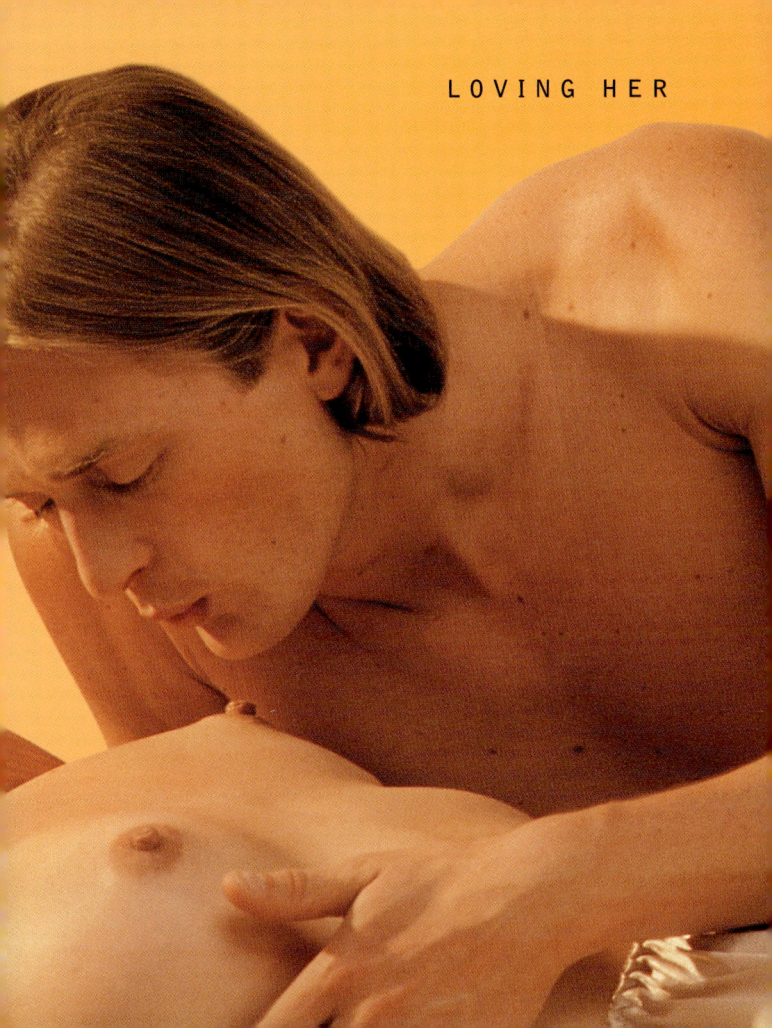

LOVING HER

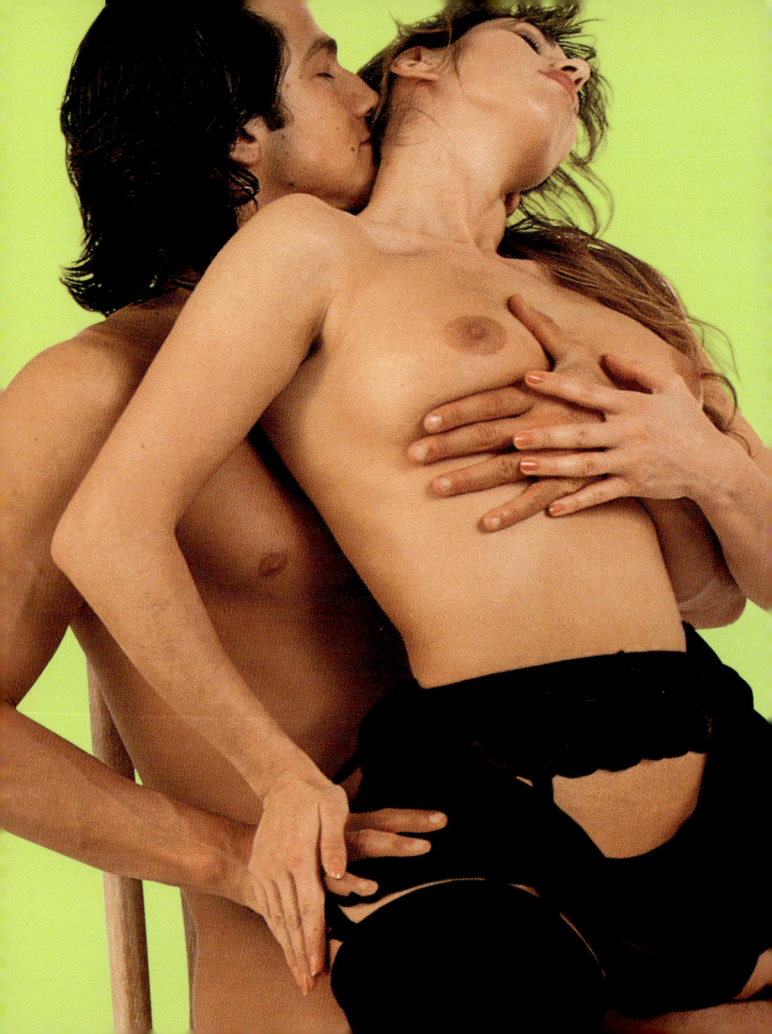

LOVING HER

ELONGATED
ORGASM

❤ Arousal takes place in the mind as well as the genitals, so whisper erotic secrets in her ear when she's close to climaxing.

❤ Maximize stimulation on her clitoris — for example, let her stimulate herself while you lick her clitoris with your tongue.

❤ Try the peaking technique on her. You let her reach mini-peaks of climax by stopping and starting stimulation, then you let her go for the big one.

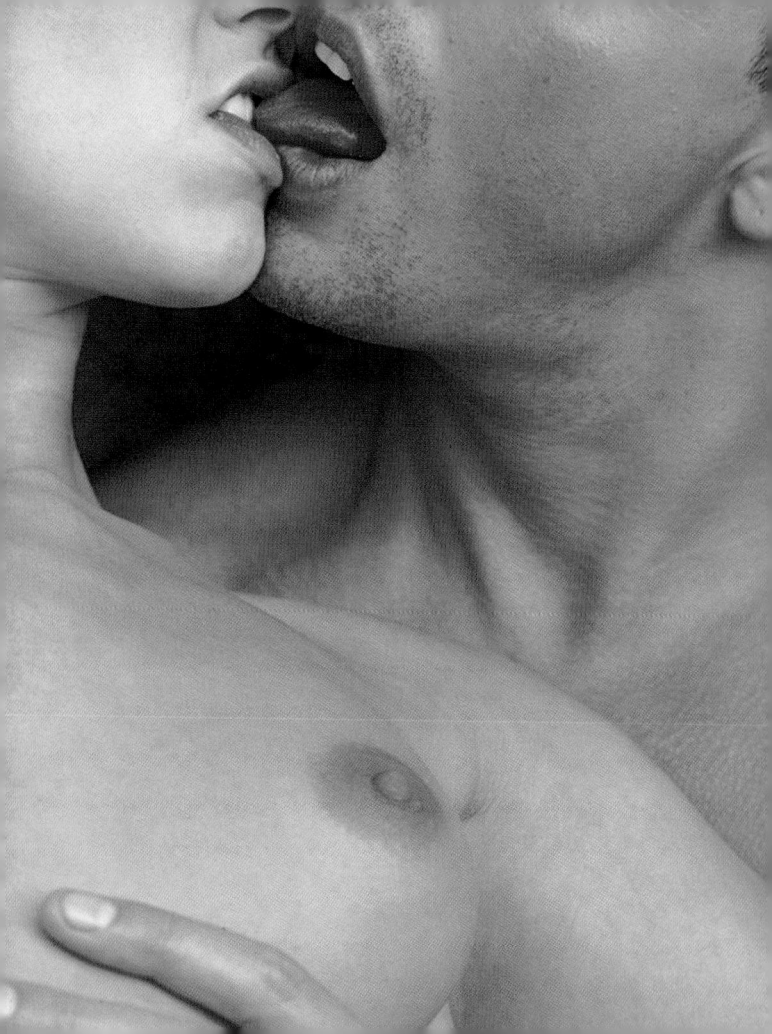

ROUGH SEX

❤ Take her by surprise with the strength of your desire. Be physically dominant – a fast, rough romp in which you take charge can be as exciting as an hour of gentle lovemaking.

❤ Always gauge her mood – if she's reluctant, back off. And – needless to say – pain and coercion are never sexy.

LOVING HER

PUSH-UPS

❤ Show her how fit you are. Do naked push-ups while your lover lies beneath you. Then penetrate her as your final exercise. Who says the missionary position is boring!

❤ Before making love to her in this position, place a couple of pillows beneath her buttocks. This raises her hips and lets her feel deeply penetrated.

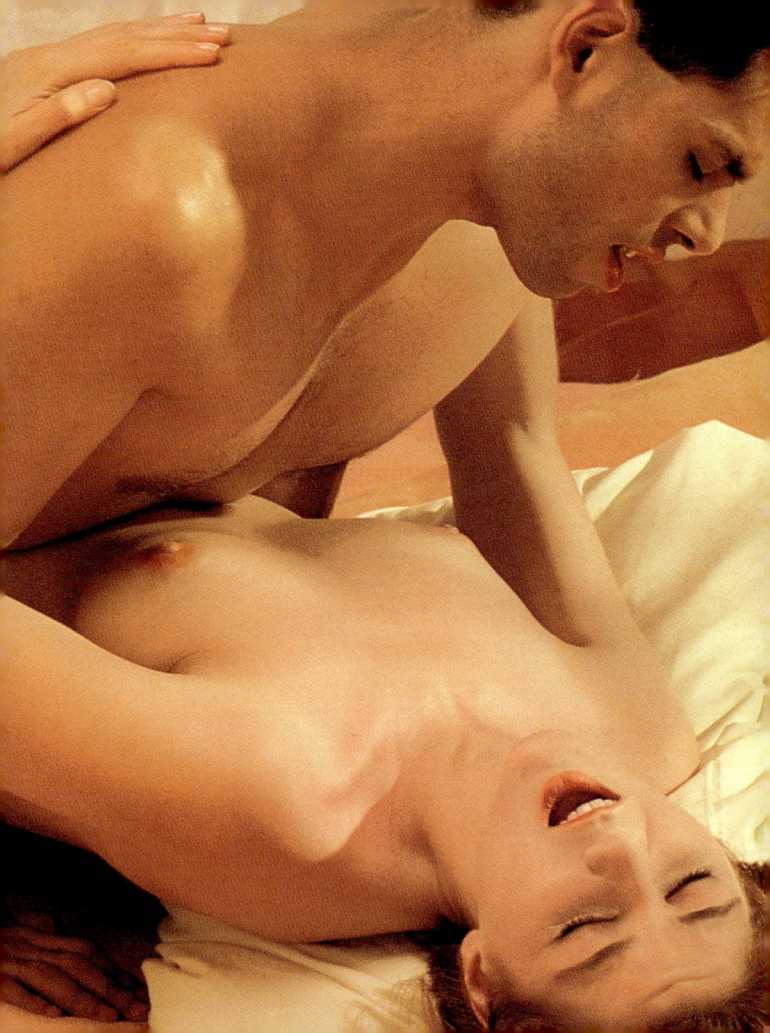

LOVING HER

INCREASING
FRICTION

❤ Fast friction on the clitoris during sex is the ultimate turn-on. Instead of thrusting, use the grind technique – stay deep inside her, and grind up and down and around.

❤ Make love in the missionary position with her legs closed so that your penis brushes her clitoris as you thrust.

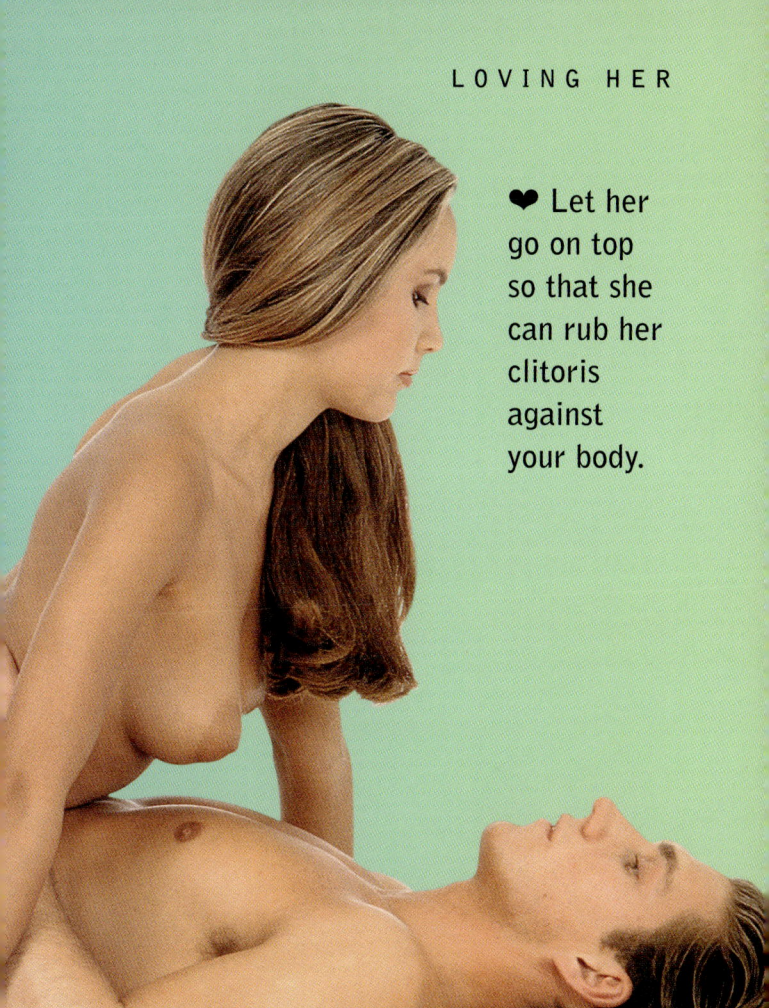

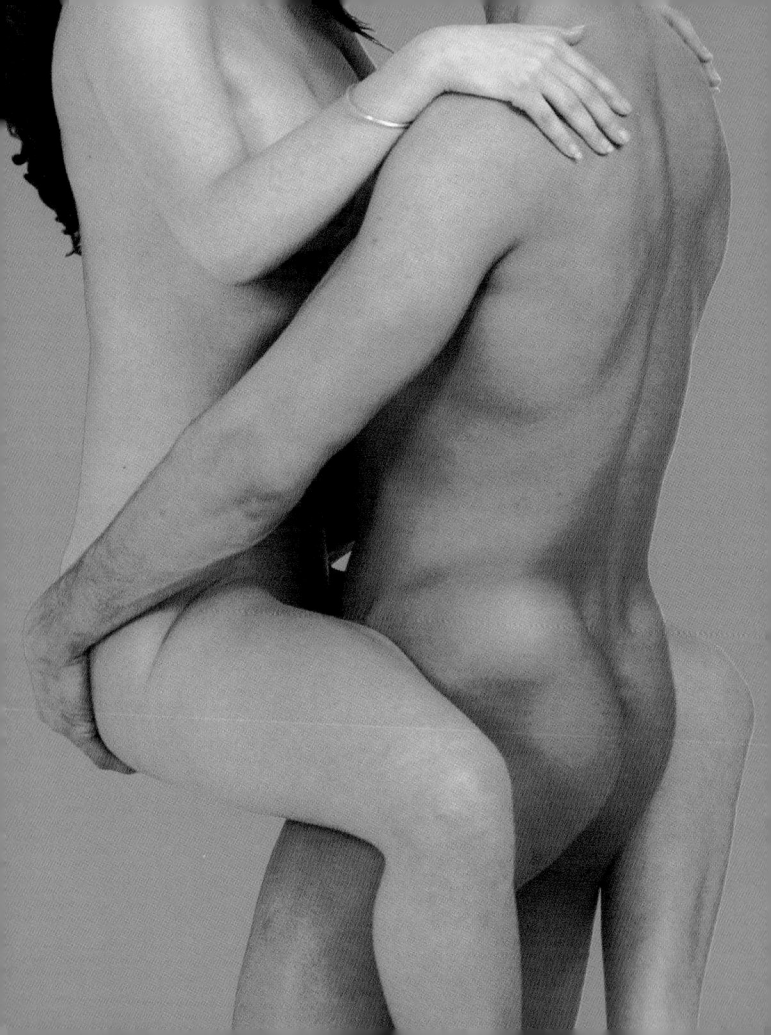

LOVING HER

AGAINST THE
WALL

❤ Spontaneous sex up against the wall shows your lover that you can't wait a moment longer to make love to her.

❤ If you can't lift her up, get her to raise one leg and bend her knee around your hip.

❤ Get her to place her hands against the wall and bend over. You penetrate her from behind, you're in such a hurry.

LOVING HER

POSITION
X-RATED

❤ Surprise her with an unusual sex position — lie on your back, bring your knees to your chest, and let her sink down onto your penis.

❤ Have a laugh with the wheelbarrow — she balances on her lower arms and elbows while you hold her legs and penetrate her.

❤ Kneel down on the floor, sit on your heels, and lean back, taking your weight on your hands. Now let her make love to you.

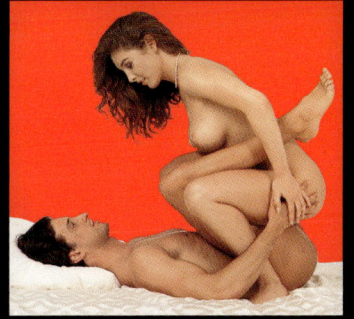

❤ Lie on your back and invite your lover to get on top – facing away from you.

❤ If you've got a large penis, lie facing your lover on your side. Get her to rest her upper thigh on your hip and then make love.

❤ If you've got a short penis, get her to lie on her front with a couple of pillows underneath her hips. Now penetrate her from behind.

LOVING HER

SPINE
TINGLER

❤ Make her tingle all over by giving her a surprise passionate kiss when you're out together in public.

❤ Send shivers down her spine by nibbling her neck and earlobes.

❤ When she's lying on her front, use your finger to trace a single line from the crown of her head down the length of her spine, over her buttocks and, finally, let it come to rest between her legs.

LOVING HER

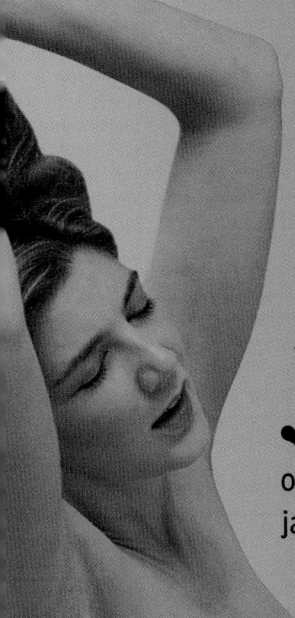

❤ Use your fingertips to make small featherlight swirls on her abdomen. Move closer and closer to her pubic hair and then back up to her navel.

❤ Give her tiny kisses on her closed eyelids, her jawline, and down the length of her spine.

❤ Kiss the soles of her feet.

❤ Massage her with a silk scarf or feather.

LOVING HER

SERIAL
CLIMAX

❤ Find out whether your woman is the serial kind by continuing to stimulate her clitoris after orgasm. If she enjoys it, keep going, and see if you can make her come again.

❤ If her clitoris is too sensitive after orgasm, spend half a minute stroking the inside of her vagina until her orgasmic contractions have died away. Now go back to her clitoris.

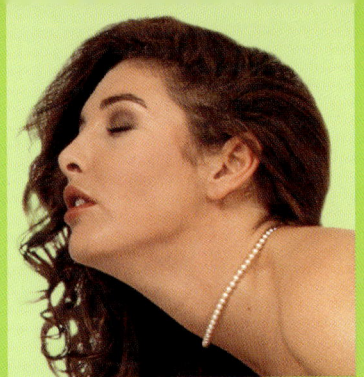

❤ Go for serial climax at times when you know her sex drive is high – when she's ovulating, or just before or during her period. And if you don't know – ask her.

❤ For a multiple treat, give her an oral sex orgasm before you have sex. Then touch her clitoris as you make love.

❤ Try not to put her under pressure to have lots of orgasms.

LOVING HER

HONEY POT

❤ Drizzle warm honey over her. Let it trickle down her chest and nipples before you lick it off.

❤ Make a honey trail from navel to clitoris. Dip your tongue into her navel and let your mouth travel slowly and tantalizingly down her body.

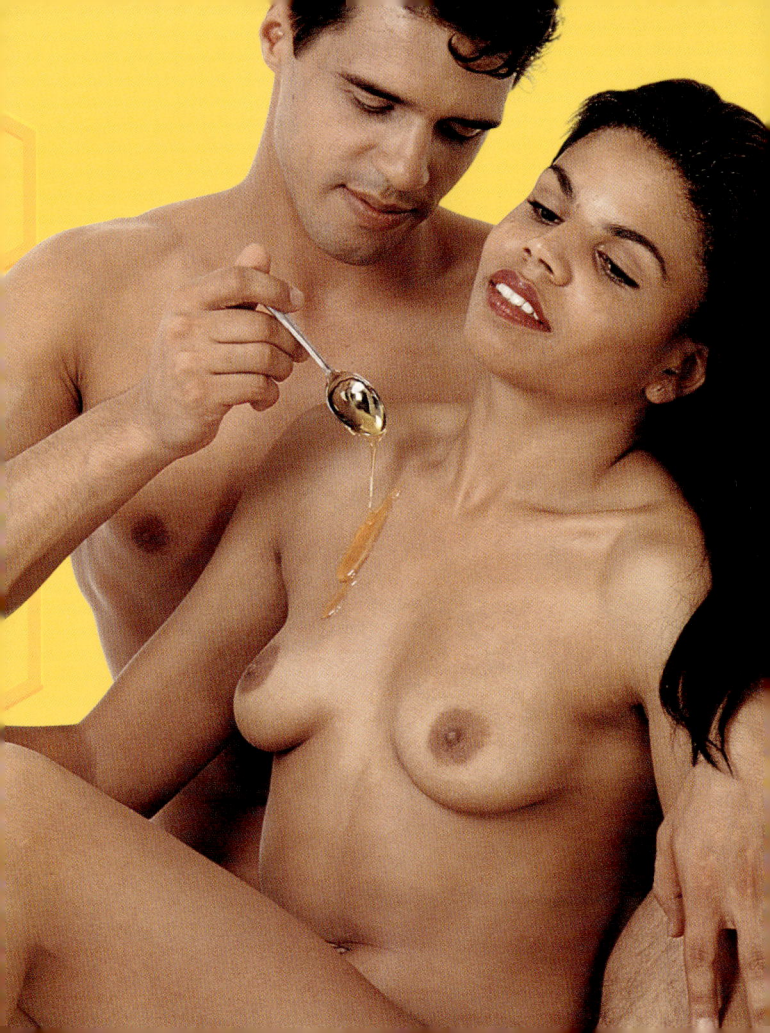

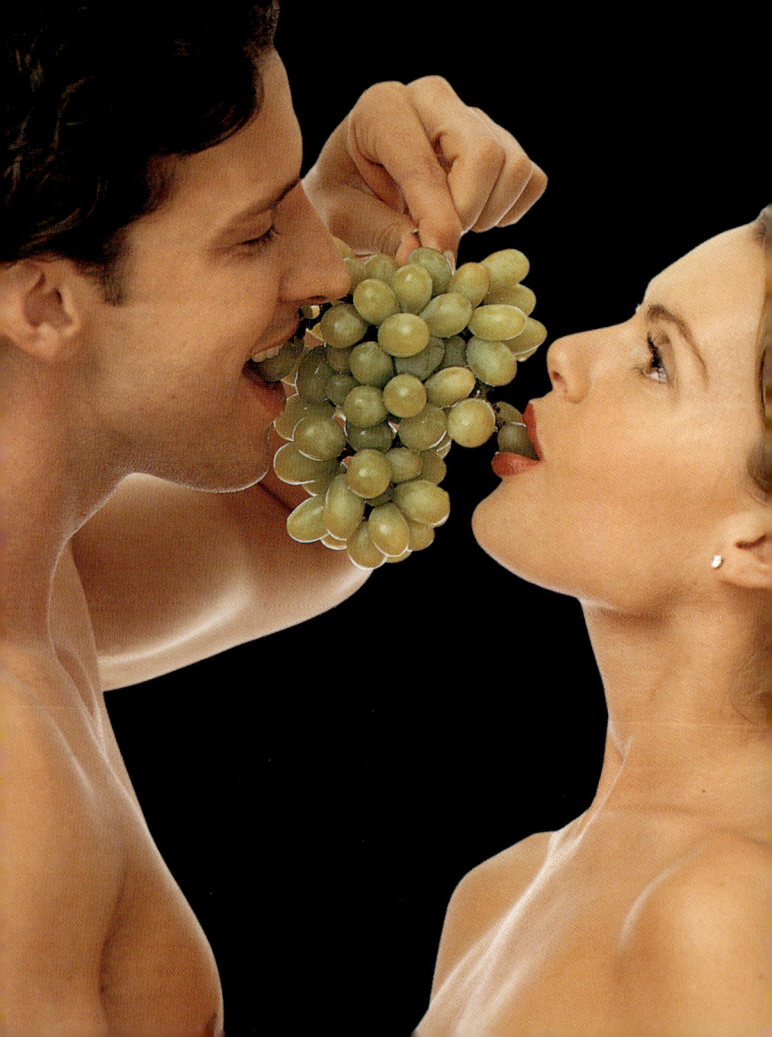

MIDNIGHT FEAST

❤ Indulge in an under-the-cover midnight feast. Feed each other grapes, and strawberries and cream with your fingers.

❤ When you're full, find other things to do with your feast. Squeeze grape juice onto her skin, crush a strawberry on her genitals and suck it off. Arrange peaks of cream on her nipples.

❤ Tickle her nipples with frozen grapes.

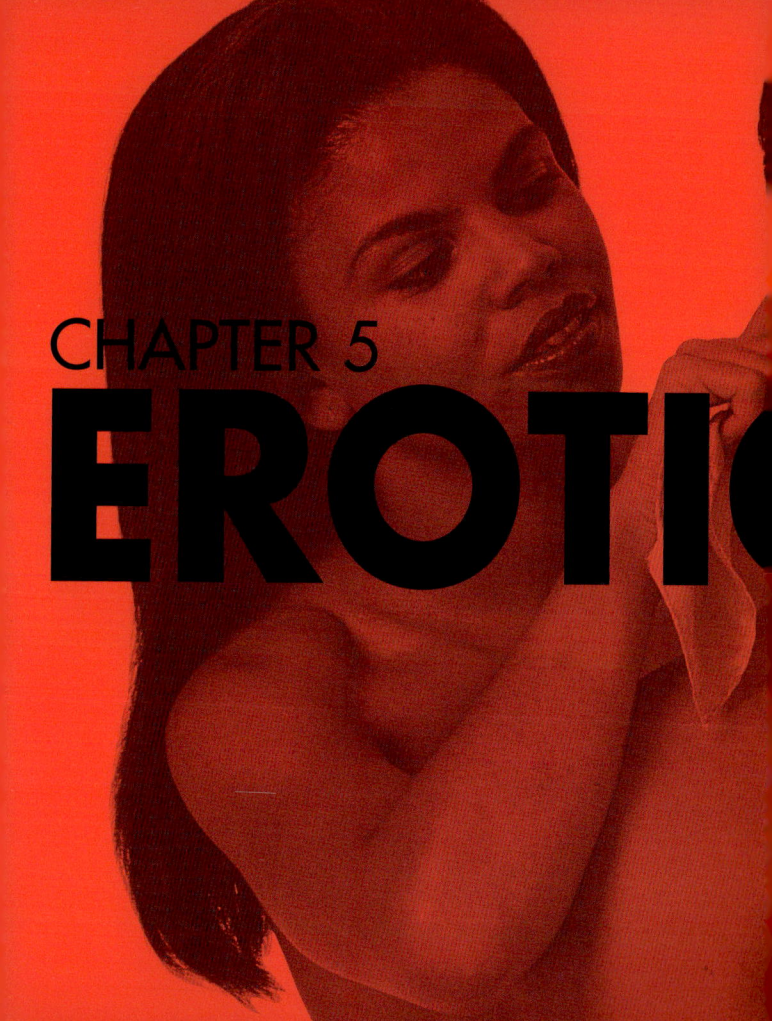
CHAPTER 5
EROTIC

TOYS

EROTIC TOYS

SEX
SHOP

❤ Plan a shopping spree with a twist: you and your partner are only allowed to buy erotica.

❤ Get ideas for your naughty purchases from sex store catalogs.

❤ If sex shops don't appeal to you, go to more traditional stores or go shopping on the internet together: www.goodvibes.com is a good start.

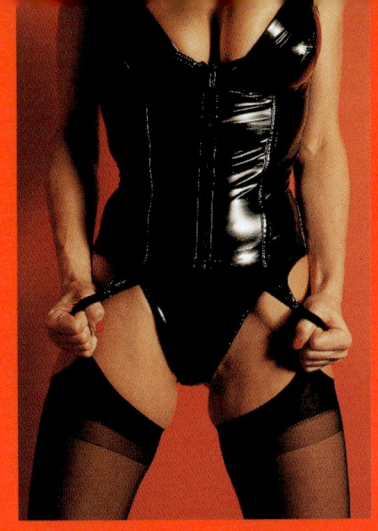

❤ Lie in bed with your lover and make a saucy shopping list: sexy lingerie, novelty condoms, flavored lubricant, a vibrator with a range of attachments ... whatever takes your interest.

❤ Take turns unwrapping all your packages – in bed.

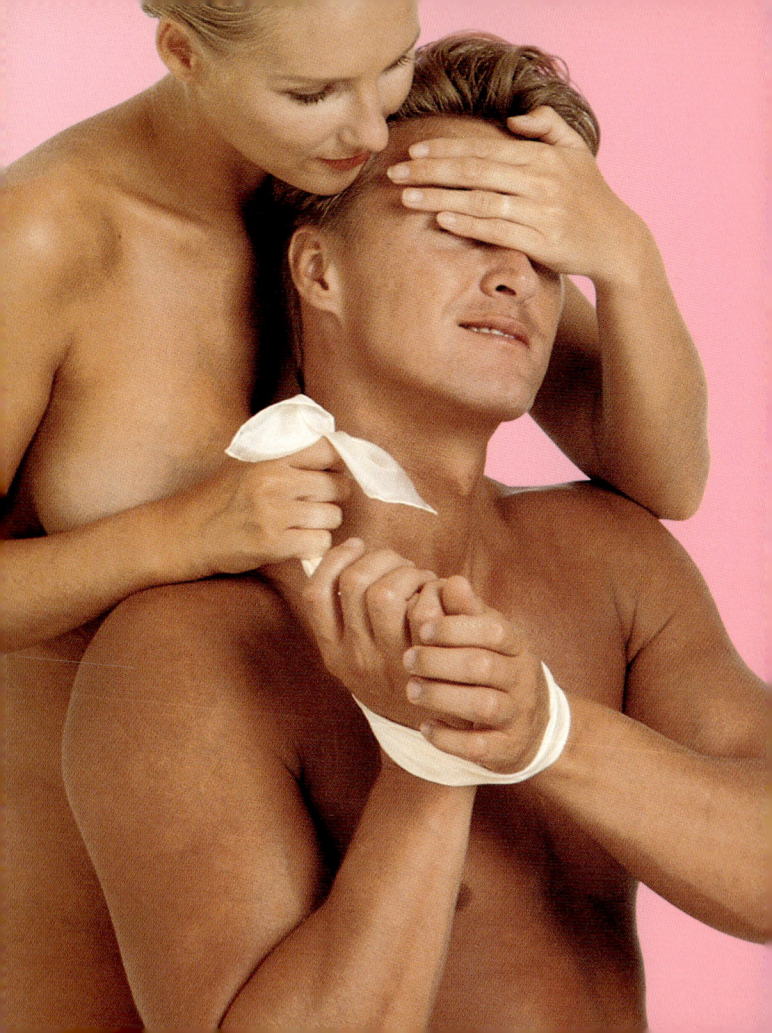

EROTIC TOYS

TOY
BOX

❤ Buy or make your own sex toy box to go under the bed. Paint it black and keep it locked – only you and your partner know where the key is kept.

❤ If your toys are really x-rated, use a box with a combination lock.

❤ Blindfold your partner and let them make their choice. Put in occasional surprises.

EROTIC TOYS

❤ Put sensual toys in your box: feathers or squares of satin, silk, fur, and velvet that you can use to caress your lover's skin.

❤ Include a book of erotic stories or fantasies that you can read aloud to each other. Or a **Kama Sutra**-style position guide with sexy pictures for inspiration.

❤ Stock up on the practical stuff such as condoms, lubricant, and massage oil.

❤ Keep a supply of items that are not obviously sex toys and improvise: a ribbon, a table tennis ball, a string of beads or a hairbrush, for example. Let your imagination run wild.

EROTIC TOYS

❤ Have a diverse collection of sex toys such as vibrators (different sizes and shapes), dildos, penis rings, anal plugs, and nipple clamps. Include mild S&M toys such as silk cords, "safe" handcuffs, blindfolds, a paddle, a cane, and a soft cat-o'-nine tails.

❤ Have dressing-up gear for every occasion: lacy black lingerie, dominatrix gear, rubber or leather pants, schoolgirl or nurse outfits, masks, and high heels.

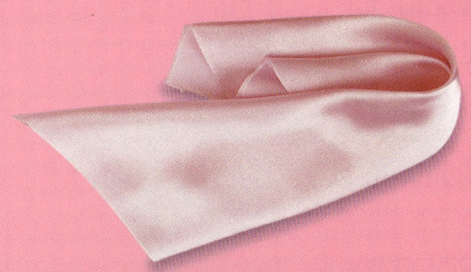

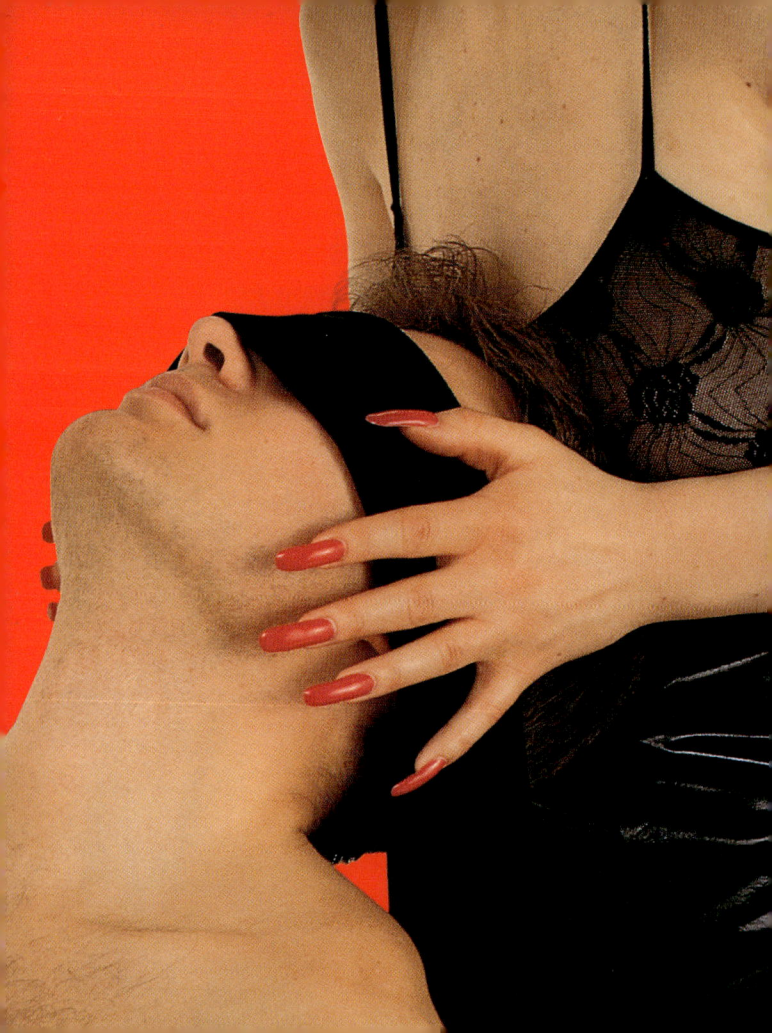

EROTIC TOYS

BLINDFOLD
BLISS

❤ The most intense titillation can arise from simply not knowing what's going to happen next – so keep your partner guessing with a blindfold.

❤ Don't make the blindfold too tight or too loose (unless peeking is part of the game). Elasticated sleeping masks are ideal.

❤ Do stuff you're normally inhibited about!

EROTIC TOYS

RUBBER
UNDIES

❤ Rubber is sexy because it shows off every single bodily curve – exploit this by wearing the tightest garments possible. Remember – loose rubber just isn't a turn on!

❤ Sprinkle talcum powder on your skin first to make your rubber undies glide on in seconds.

❤ Don't use oil on rubber – it damages it.

EROTIC TOYS

❤ Wear a rubber catsuit and get your partner to spray you down with special rubber spray.

❤ Dress each other in rubber and go to nightclubs. Watch the sweat flow as the temperature rises.

❤ Throw a fetish party: latex shorts, vests, and bodysuits for the boys; latex stockings, corsets, and dresses for the girls.

❤ Choose rubberwear that allows fast access to the important parts — crotch zippers or lace-up bodices, for example.

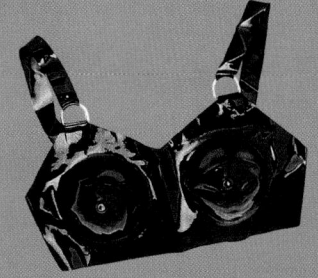

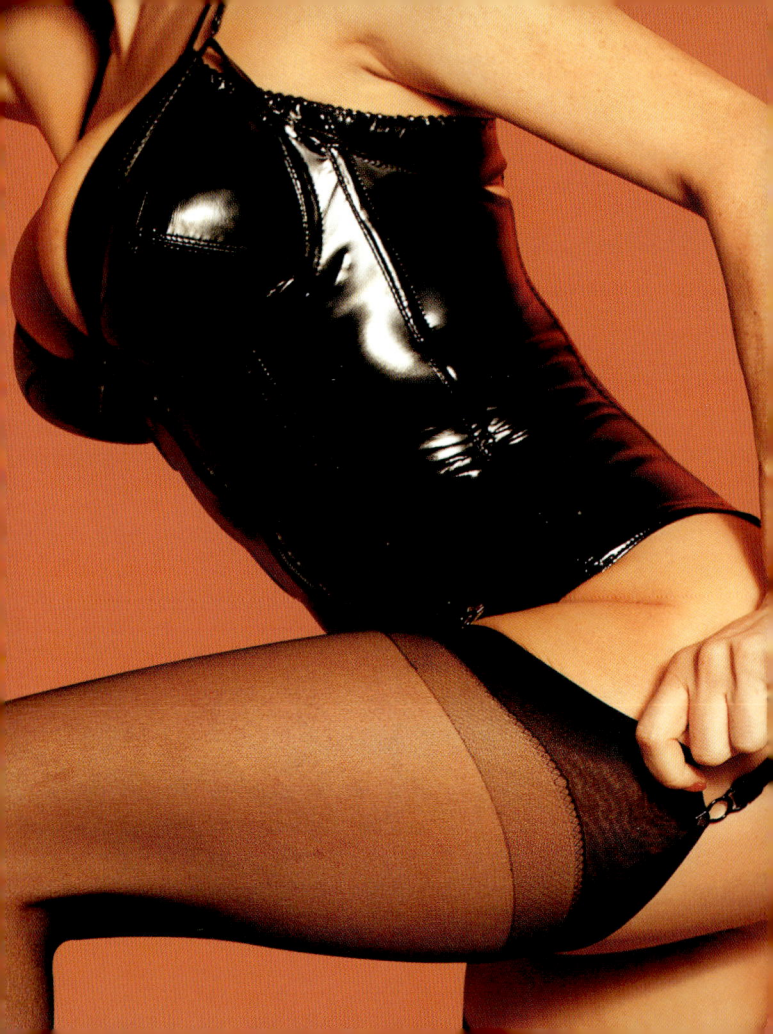

EROTIC TOYS

LEATHER AND
MASKS

❤ Make sex sizzle by dressing up in black and red leather. If it smells strong, so much the better.

❤ So that your partner feels that he or she is being treated to a new experience, make sure you wear a mask – it offers erotic disguise.

❤ Be inventive with leather belts – use them to restrain each other.

EROTIC TOYS

SATIN AND LACE

❤ Go for a sexy but virginal look with pure white satin garters and panties, and sheer stockings with lacy tops.

❤ Give your partner a genital massage while wearing a pair of lacy gloves.

❤ Turn your bedroom into a romantic haven, with satin sheets and pillow cases sprayed with your favorite perfume.

❤ Stroke every inch of your partner's skin with pieces of velvet, satin, silk, and lace. You can brush the fabrics across the main part of his body to tickle and tease. Only toward the end should your stroking focus on the genitals.

❤ For a soft-core bondage experience, blindfold him with satin, and bind his wrists together with lace.

❤ Titillate your partner by wearing a transparent lace dress.

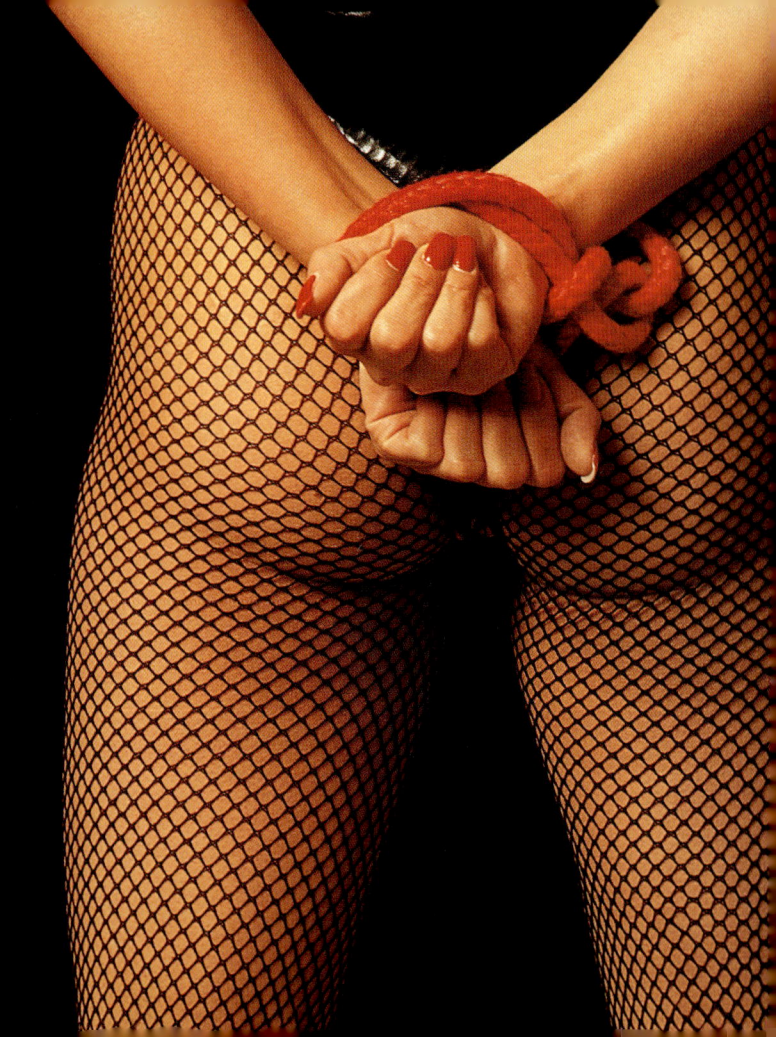

EROTIC TOYS

BONDAGE
BABE

❤ Wear bondage gear – walk him around on a leather leash, bind her wrists with cord, carry a leather whip by your side, or chain yourself to each other. Be strict!

❤ Wear a spanking skirt that reveals your buttocks, or a keyhole dress that shows off your breasts.

❤ Agree a code word that means "stop."

EROTIC TOYS

GOOD
VIBES

❤ Many women find the fast and powerful oscillations produced by a vibrator are the most reliable way to reach orgasm, both on

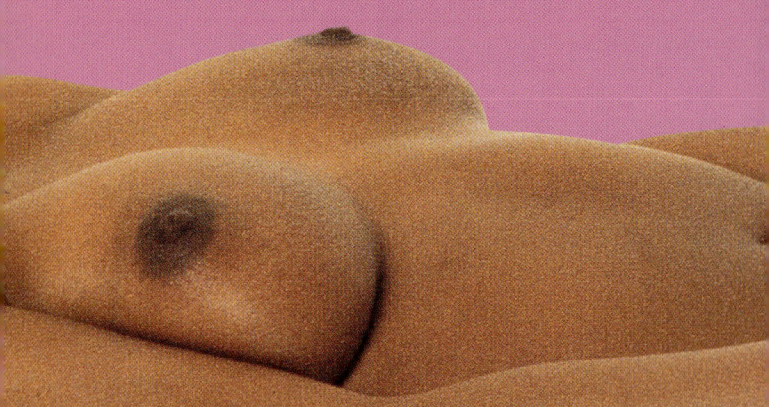

EROTIC TOYS

their own and during sex with a partner. If you've never used a vibrator, give yourself a sexual treat and try one now!

❤ Men love vibrators too. Experiment by holding one against the head and shaft of the penis, and the entrance to the anus.

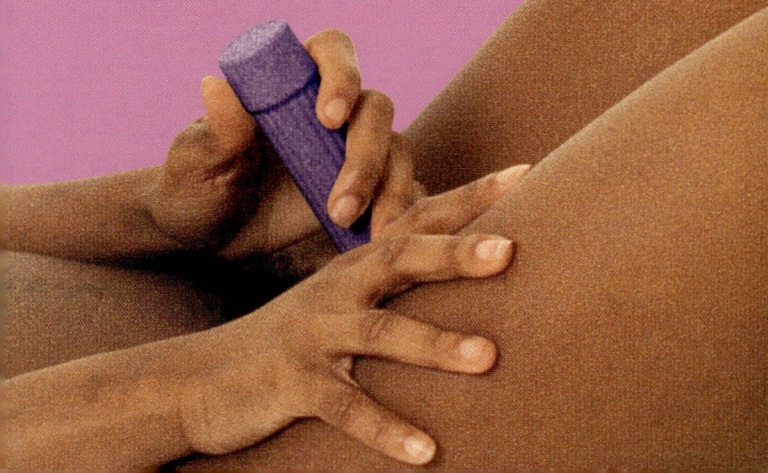

EROTIC TOYS

❤ The very latest vibrator technology is used in a new vibrator known as "natural contour," which is designed by women for women. It's purse-shaped rather than phallic, and fits neatly into a purse. Your mother wouldn't recognize it!

❤ The pocket rocket is a small flashlight-like vibrator that can be dressed in rich jelly-colored sleeves that come in different textures. Select the texture that suits you best. This vibrator may be small, but its textures ensure it does the job!

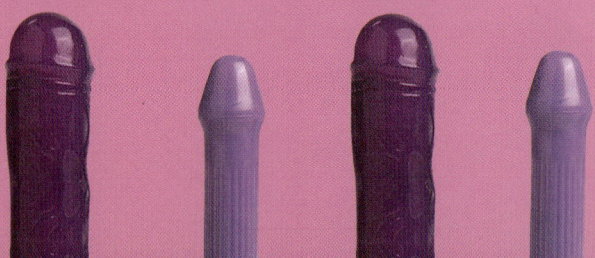

EROTIC TOYS

❤ Double the sexual sensation by using two vibrators at once – one on the clitoris and one on the vaginal entrance. Get your partner to assist.

❤ Use a vibrator to massage the whole of your and your partner's body – not just the genitals.

❤ If you notice a decline in sensation when you use your vibrator, it's probably due to fading batteries. Keep a supply of long-life batteries close at hand.

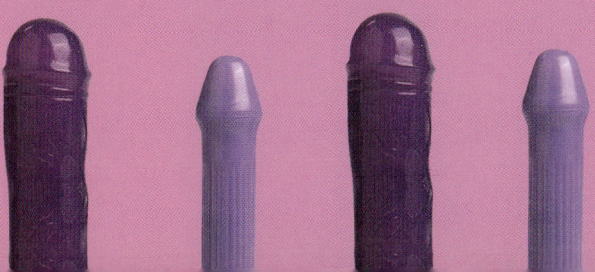

EROTIC TOYS

ITEMS AT
HAND

❤ You don't have to spend a fortune on sex toys. With the help of your imagination you can turn almost any everyday item into an erotic aid. Just avoid vacuum cleaners!

❤ Reinvent uses for the following items: a pair of rubber gloves, a feather, a large silk handkerchief, a toothbrush, a roll of bubble wrap, a rolling pin, a bottle of olive oil, a kitchen spatula, a clean paint roller, some wax candles, and a water pistol.

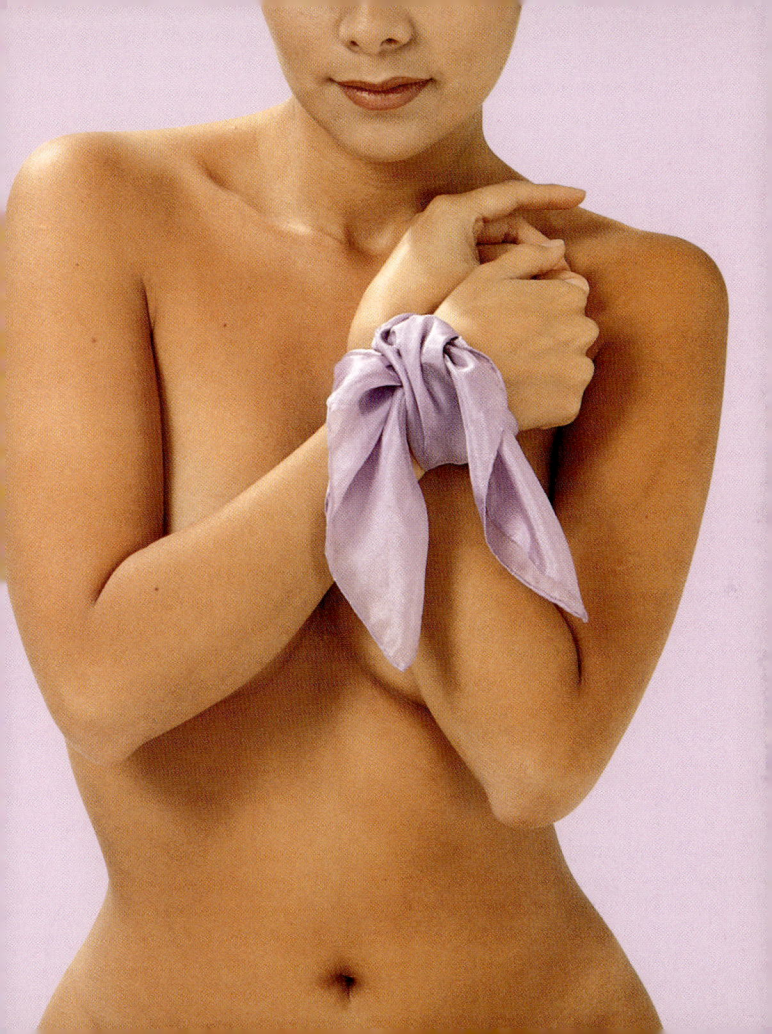

EROTIC TOYS

SPANKING
TOOLS

❤ Indulge in a buttock-tingling spanking session. Use a leather paddle (this comes in a wide flat shape that spreads neatly across the buttocks), a soft whip or flail, or a carpet beater. Hardcore spanking tools are canes, rulers, and leather whips – these hurt, so use them with caution!

❤ For on-the-spot punishment, improvise with whatever you can find – the back of your hand, a hairbrush, or a towel.

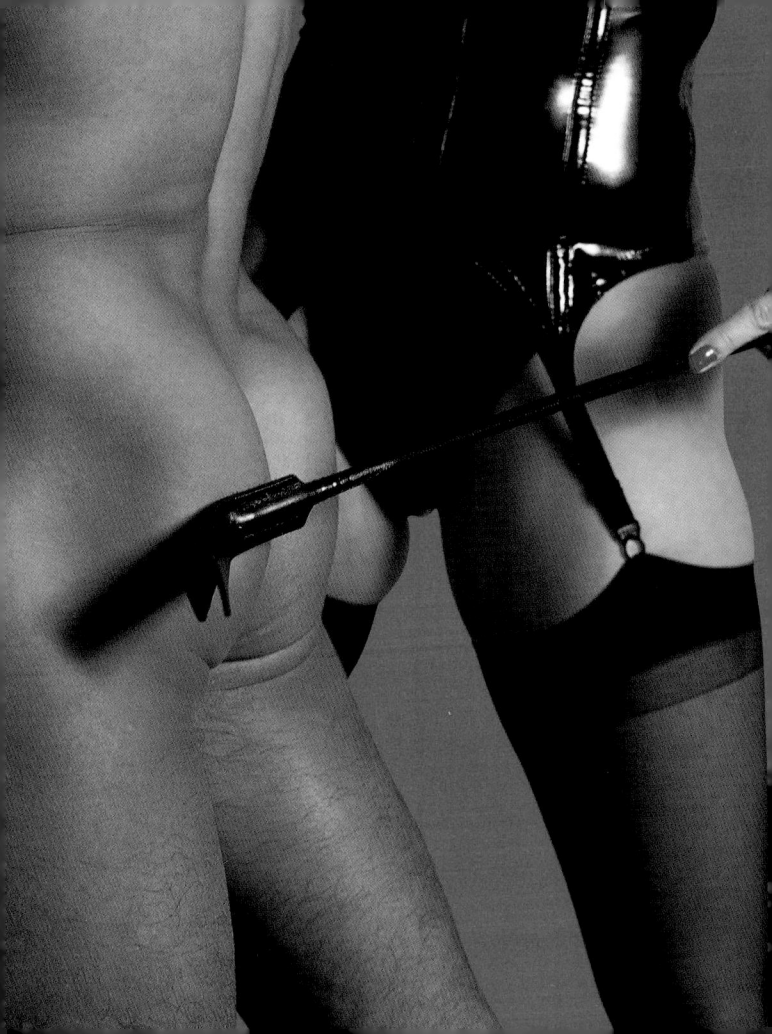

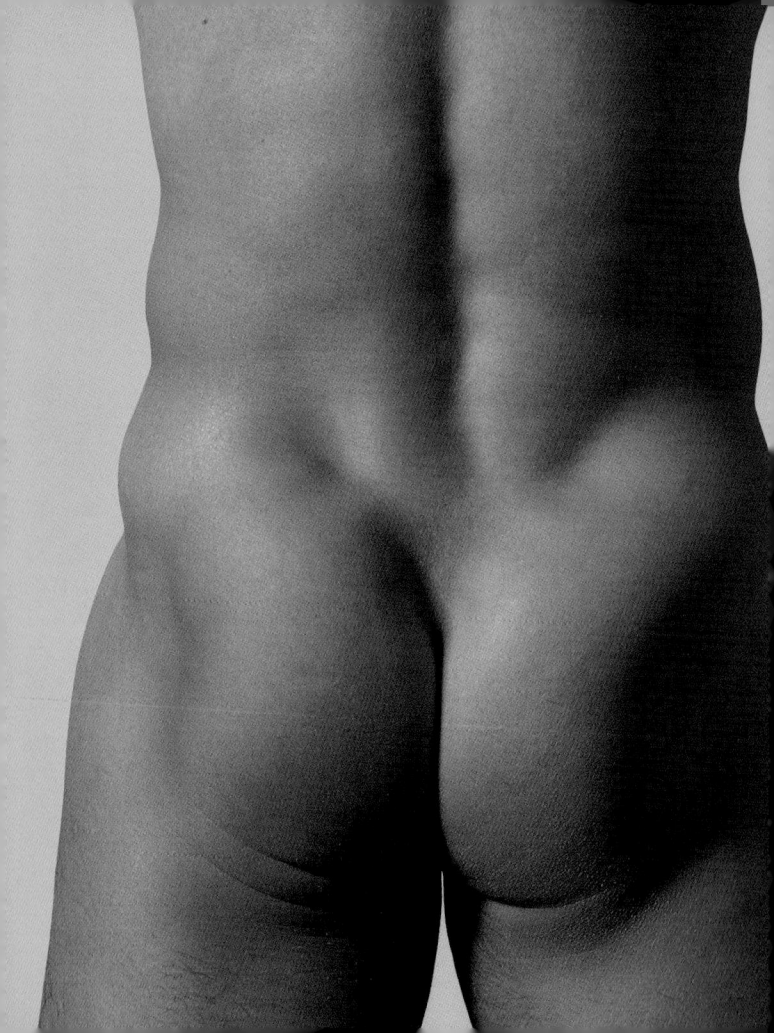

EROTIC TOYS

NOVELTY
CONDOM

❤ Condoms come in every shape, color, texture, and flavor. Have fun trying out different types, but always use a good-quality brand – and make sure that you check the use-by date.

❤ Choose ribbed and textured for her pleasure, and ultrathin for his pleasure.

❤ When you know her better, find some wildly colored sheaths that you wear in bed for fun!

EROTIC TOYS

FLAVORING
FUN

❤ Paint each other's nipples with warm melted chocolate.

❤ Give your partner oral sex while sucking a mentholated candy.

❤ Make ice cubes from exotic fruit juice, such as mango and passion fruit. Melt the ice on your lover's body. Now lick!

EROTIC TOYS

❤ Recent sex store successes are fruit lubes. These are lubricants in gelatine-capsule form. Pop one in your mouth before oral sex and bite on it as you engulf your lover. The lube floods your mouth in wonderful fruit flavors, and assists your loving mouth massage.

❤ Put on loads of glossy, slippery lip gloss on and make your lover kiss it off.

❤ Have sticky fun by using honey or syrup instead of a lubricant.

❤ Squeeze soft fruits over each other's bodies and lick the juice and pulp off before making love.

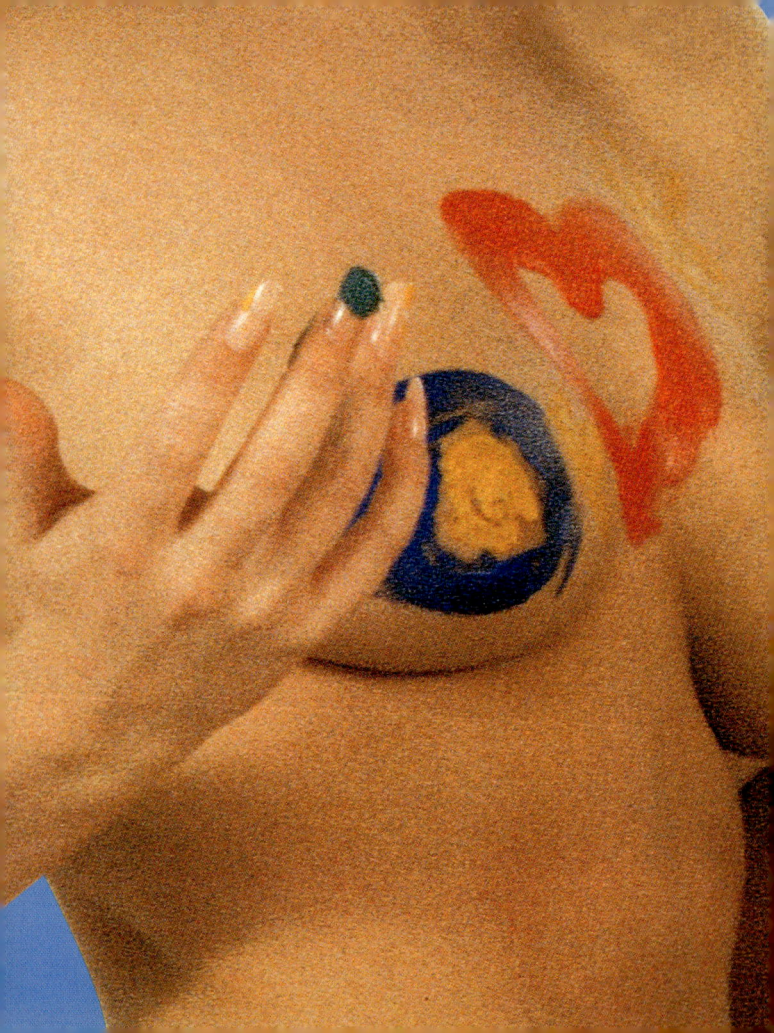

EROTIC TOYS

BRUSH
STROKES

❤ Treat your partner to an x-rated painting class. Lay her down on a towel and carefully color in all her special erogenous zones with face paint (or an edible "paint," such as cream). Don't forget to flick your paintbrush as tantalizingly as possible.

❤ Arrange your partner in a provocative position on the bed and sketch his naked body. No touching until your drawing is complete.

EROTIC TOYS

FRUIT AND
VEG

❤ Cut a pineapple ring to fit exactly around his penis. Then nibble it off.

❤ Use phallic-shaped vegetables, such as carrots or cucumbers, as natural dildos.

❤ Mash peaches and papaya together to create a deliciously fruity and edible genital lubricant.

EROTIC TOYS

❤ Masturbate with a fruit-flavored ice-lolly prior to oral sex.

❤ Cover each other in watermelon flesh.

❤ Decorate his penis with strawberries and cream. Now take a polaroid!

❤ Show him how you plan to give oral sex – on a banana!

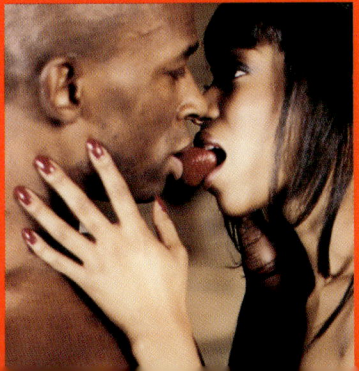

CHAPTER
SEX

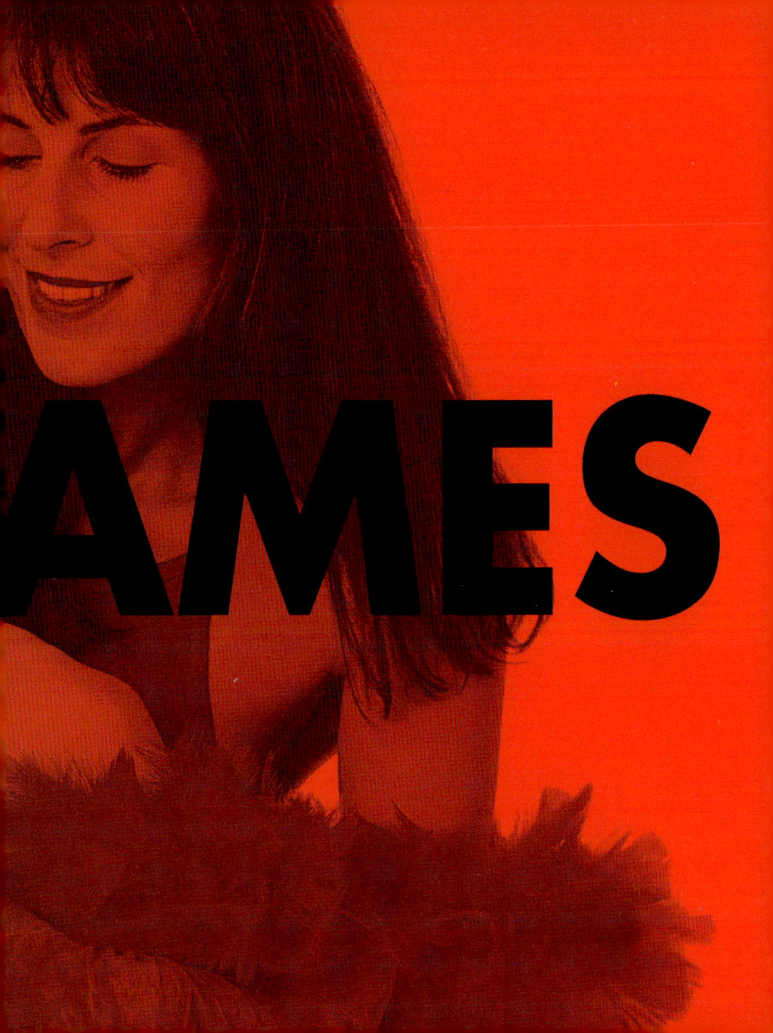

SEX GAMES

ADULT
PLAY

♥ Turn up the sexual tension by playing naughty role-playing games with your lover. Agree in advance what you will and won't do and that the game can stop on request.

♥ The best fantasy games are those in which you behave completely in character. So dress up in costumes or masks, buy props and toys – use your imagination, and do whatever it takes.

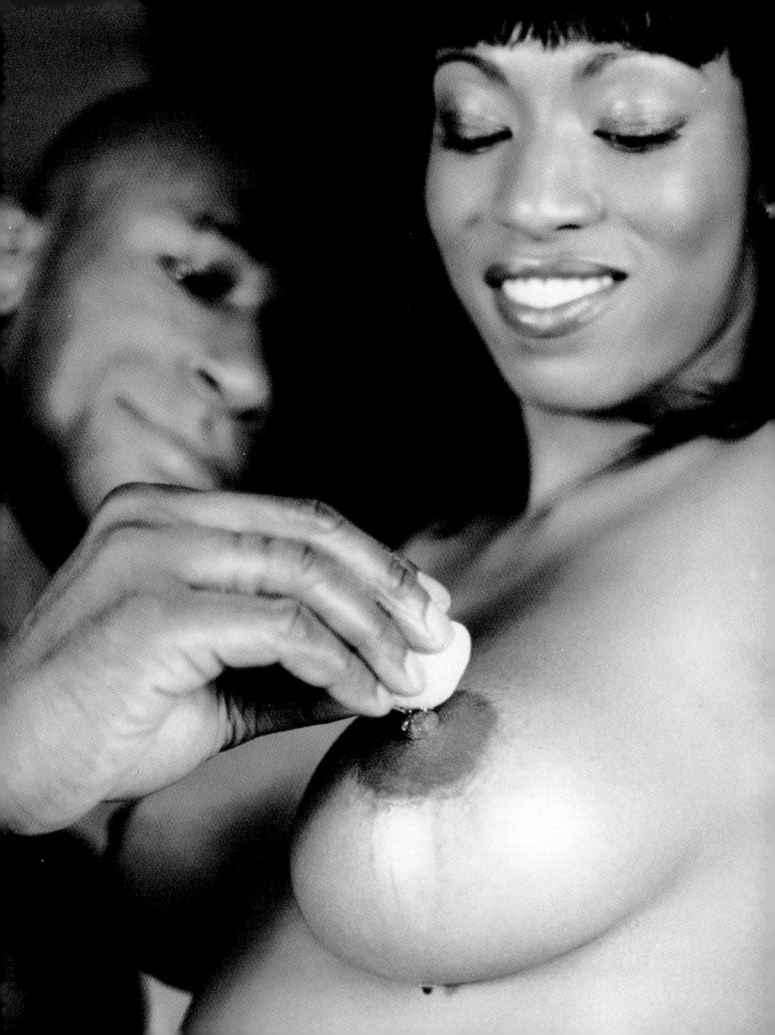

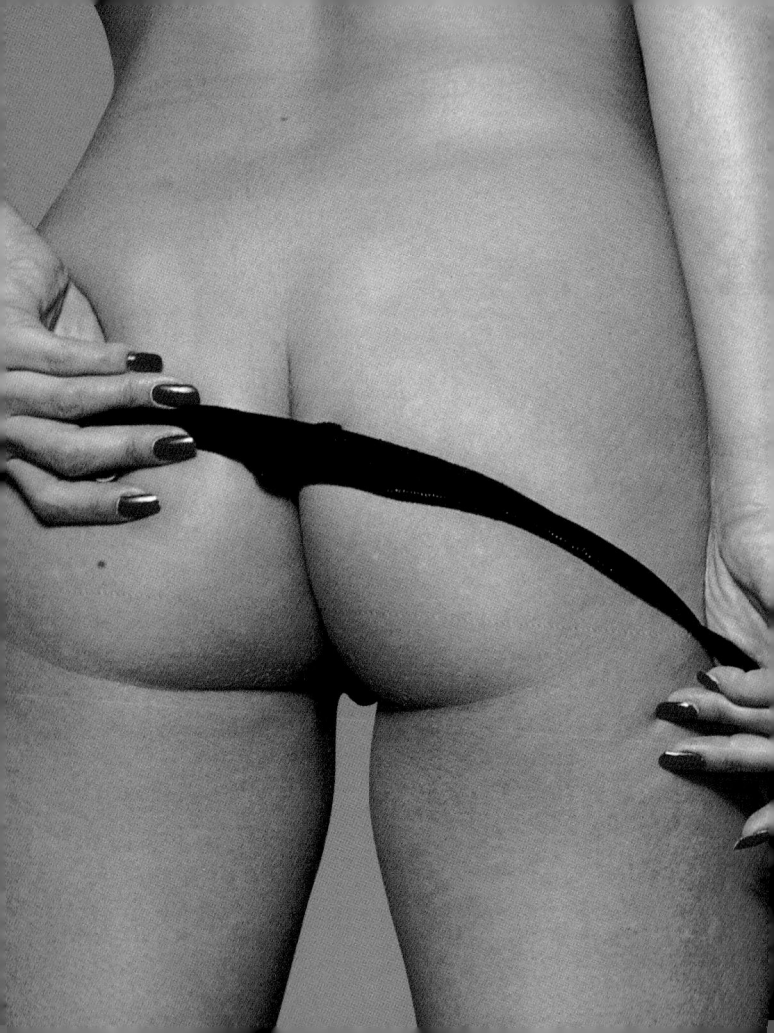

SEX GAMES

TREASURE
HUNT

❤ Tease your lover with an envelope containing a written clue. For example, "if you want to make love tonight, look in your top drawer." This clue leads to another and another until your lover is led to a sexy surprise, such as a sex toy (together with instructions from you about how you think it should be used), or you lying in bed clad in nothing more than your sexiest underwear and fragrance.

SEX GAMES

CHAIN
GANG

❤ Punish your partner for being bad – make them wear a collar, and chain them to the bed.

❤ Tantalize your partner with provocative glimpses of your body or stimulation that stops and starts without warning.

❤ Tell your partner that if they moves you will cane them. Then cane them anyway!

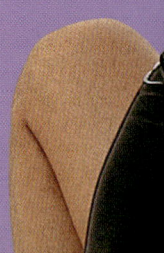

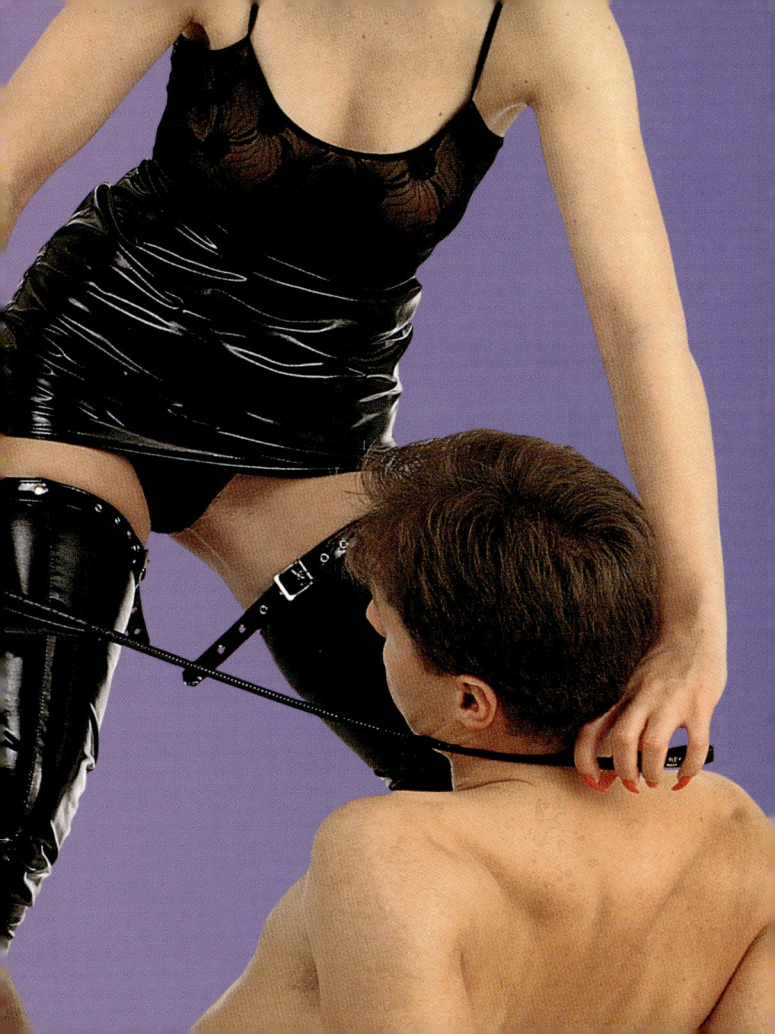

SEX GAMES

HONEYMOON
AGAIN

❤ Reserve a room at a small hotel for the weekend, preferably surrounded by beautiful countryside – make sure that no one can contact you. Leave your mobile phone at home or switch it off.

❤ Don't talk about work or domestic issues – leave your day-to-day life behind.

❤ Act out your fantasy of perfect honeymoon sex.

SEX GAMES

❤ Spend time rediscovering each other – go for long walks, share slow, seductive baths in flickering candlelight, and spend a long time lying in bed touching each other.

❤ Be romantic: hold hands, make lots of eye contact, tell each other how much you love each other, and buy each other little presents that will act as mementoes of your weekend.

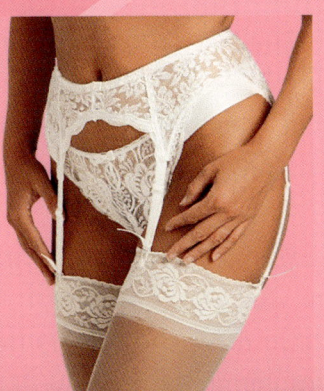

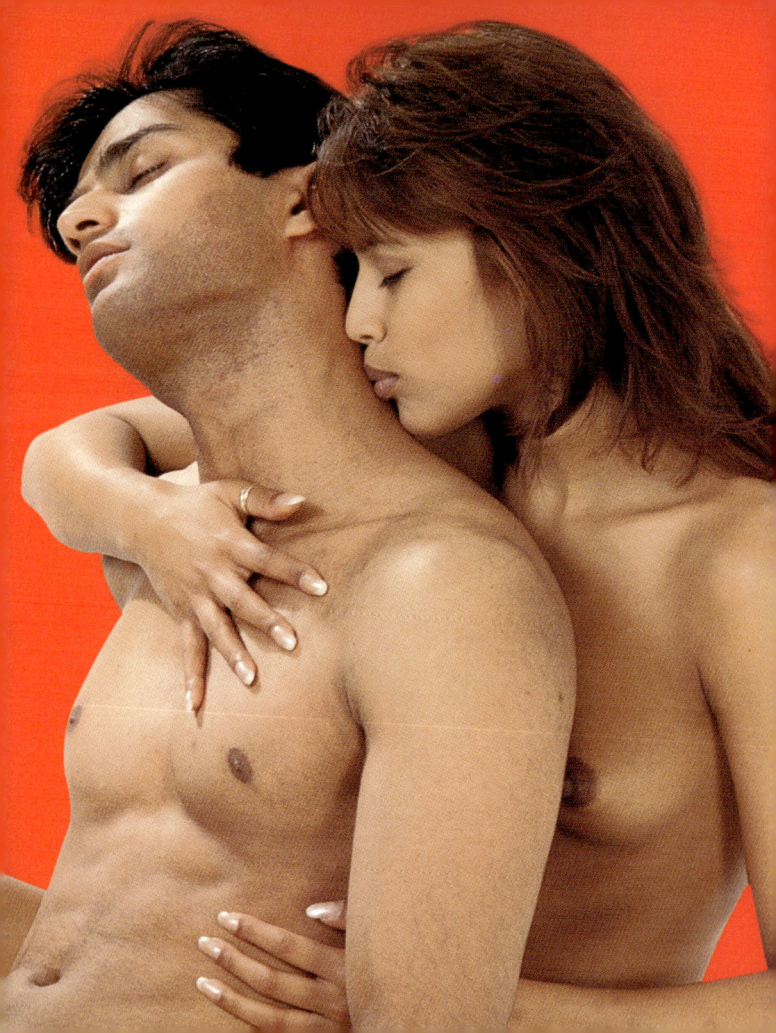

SEX GAMES

KISSES AND
BITES

❤ Spend 15 minutes kissing – nothing else.

❤ Change your kissing style – if you're normally a passionate kisser, try being restrained and reserved.

❤ Bite down upon your partner's neck, but not enough to break the skin.

❤ French kiss each other's feet or belly.

SEX GAMES

FIRST AID

❤ Play doctor and patient by dressing up in a white coat and surgical gloves, and white gown respectively.

❤ The patient should hop up onto a table and prepare to be examined.

❤ The doctor should make a thorough examination of the erogenous zones.

SEX GAMES

❤ If the patient is female, ask her to spread her legs, and press your surgically gloved fingers around her clitoris and the entrance to her vagina.

❤ If the patient is male, conduct an in-depth examination of his penis and scrotum.

❤ As the doctor you must never reveal any signs of arousal. As you touch the patient, keep asking "And how does this feel?"

❤ As the patient, you must submit to the doctor's touch. Don't try to respond.

SEX GAMES

THE
BOSS

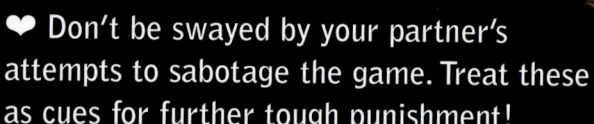

❤ Take total control of your lover during sex. Tell him or her what you want and insist on 100 percent obedience – or else!

❤ Don't be swayed by your partner's attempts to sabotage the game. Treat these as cues for further tough punishment!

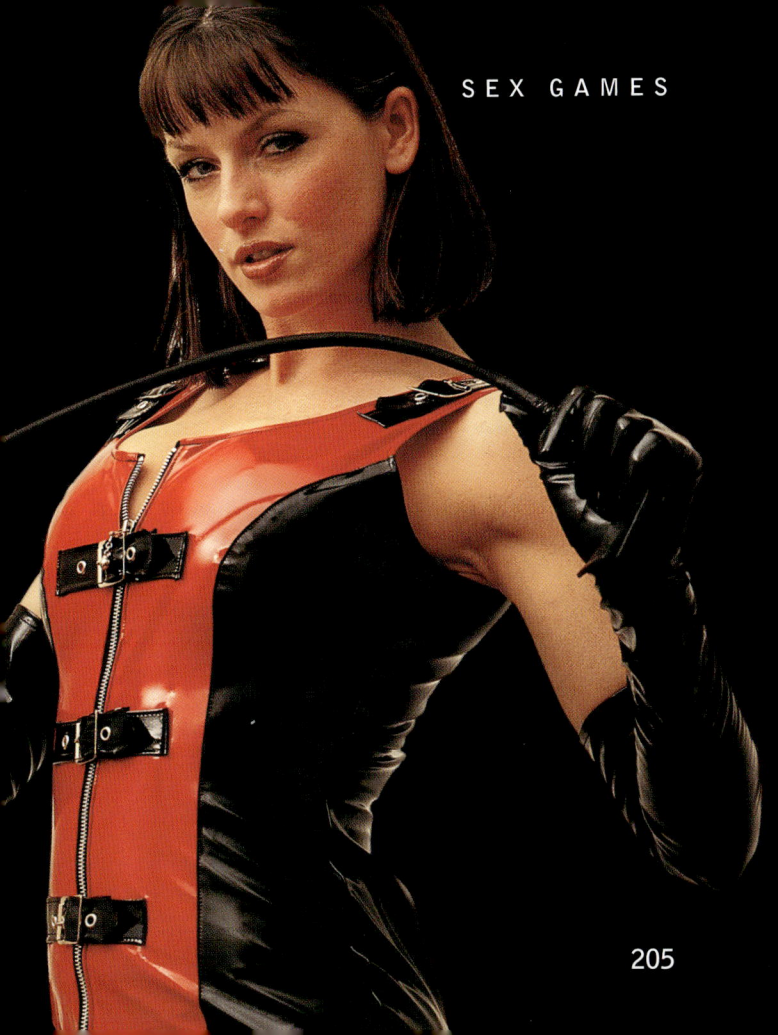

SEX GAMES

SCHOOL
DAYS

❤ Men love girls in uniform, so indulge him in his favorite fantasy – dress up in a thigh-skimming school dress and a pair of socks that end just below the hemline.

❤ Pretend that he is the sexually repressed teacher and you are the naughty schoolgirl who will liberate him.

❤ Kiss behind the gym.

SEX GAMES

❤ When your man reaches out to caress your bare legs, be shocked. Tell him he should keep his hands to himself. But at the same time sidle in closer and closer.

❤ Throw a saucy costume party with a school disco theme – the rule is you have to get off with someone by midnight.

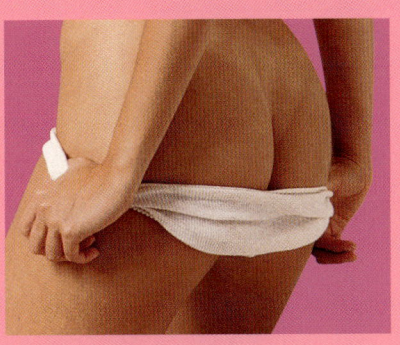

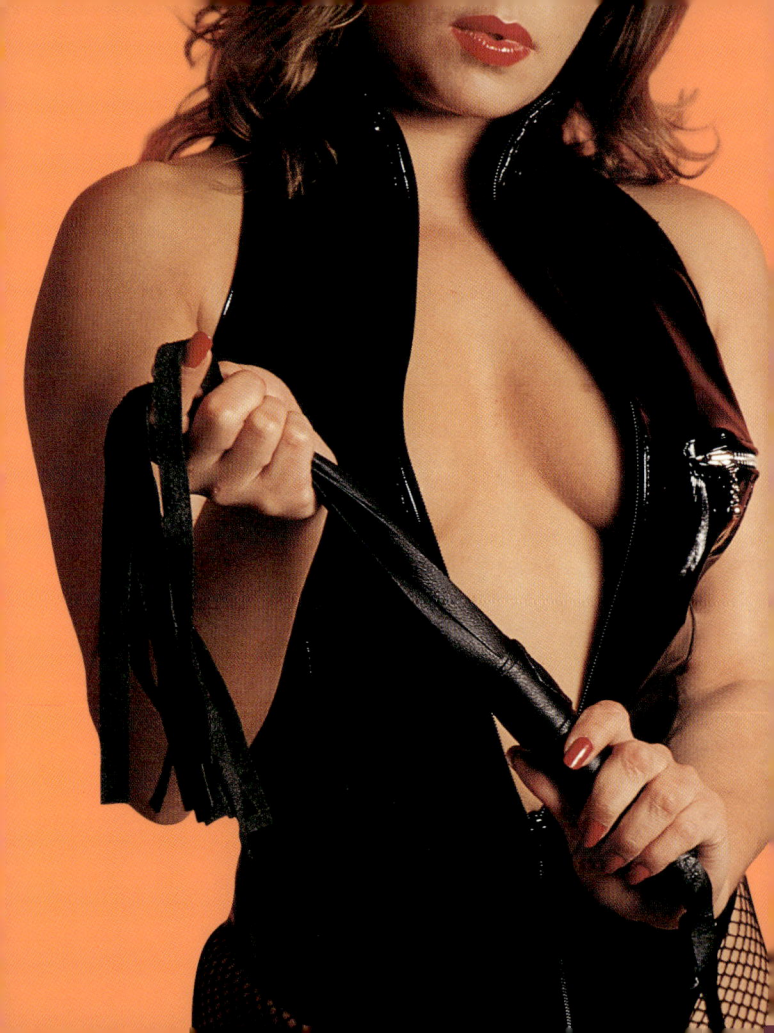

SEX GAMES

I DARE
YOU...

❤ Play truth or dare, or a card game in which the loser must carry out a task. Sexy tasks include stripping, revealing a secret erotic fantasy, or dressing up in fetish gear.

❤ Use sexual dares to take your relationship across new erotic boundaries. Dare your partner to do something that you have never tried together.

SEX GAMES

EDIBLE
SEX

♥ Think of your lover as a beautiful table upon which you arrange a small but sensual picnic. The aim of the game — to eat your way to sex!

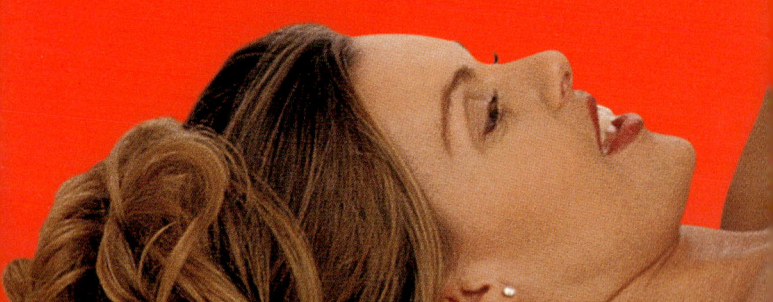

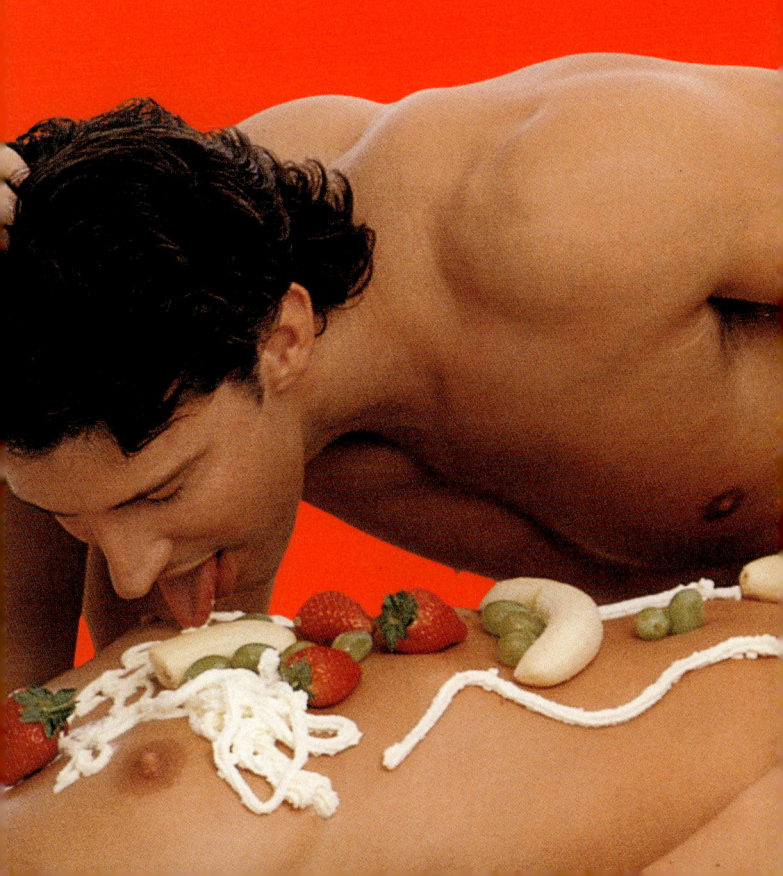

SEX GAMES

SEX GAMES

❤ Put a juicy red strawberry on the part of the body where you most want to be licked and kissed. Keep moving it!

❤ Create unbearable anticipation during dinner by presenting a written menu to your lover in advance. On the dessert section simply write: "me."

❤ Have a summer picnic in the yard by candlelight and then come indoors and make love.

❤ Re-enact the sex-in-front-of-the-fridge scene from the film **9½ Weeks**.

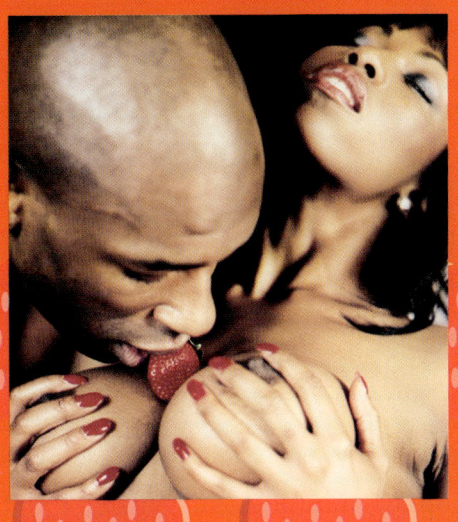

❤ Feed cherries to each other by dangling the stems from your lips.

❤ Feed buttered spaghetti to each other and let the butter trickle down your chin.

SEX GAMES

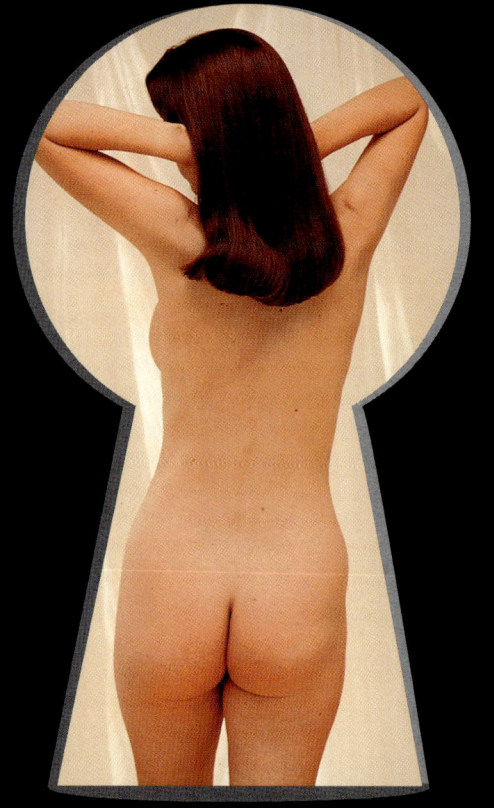

SEX GAMES

PEEP
HOLE

♥ Invite your lover to spy on you as you take a bath or shower. Make sure you put on an especially hot performance.

♥ Arrange the mirrors in your bedroom so that your partner can watch you undressing from every angle. Then invite them to lie back and enjoy the view.

SEX GAMES

FILM
STAR

♥ Dedicate a special fantasy evening to yourself and imagine that your favorite film star is coming over to make love to you.

SEX GAMES

❤ Stimulate yourself with your fantasy figure in mind.

❤ You can even extend this technique to making love with your partner – after all, there are no rules that say that you have to confess the source of your passion.

❤ Indulge your superstar fantasies by dressing celebrity-style and then making love.

SEX GAMES

WET AND
WILD

❤ Drizzle each other in liquid soap and then rub your bodies together.

❤ Stimulate each other using the fine jet of the shower head.

❤ Wash your partner's genitals, but make your cleaning routine last 10 minutes.

❤ Kiss while the water runs over your faces.

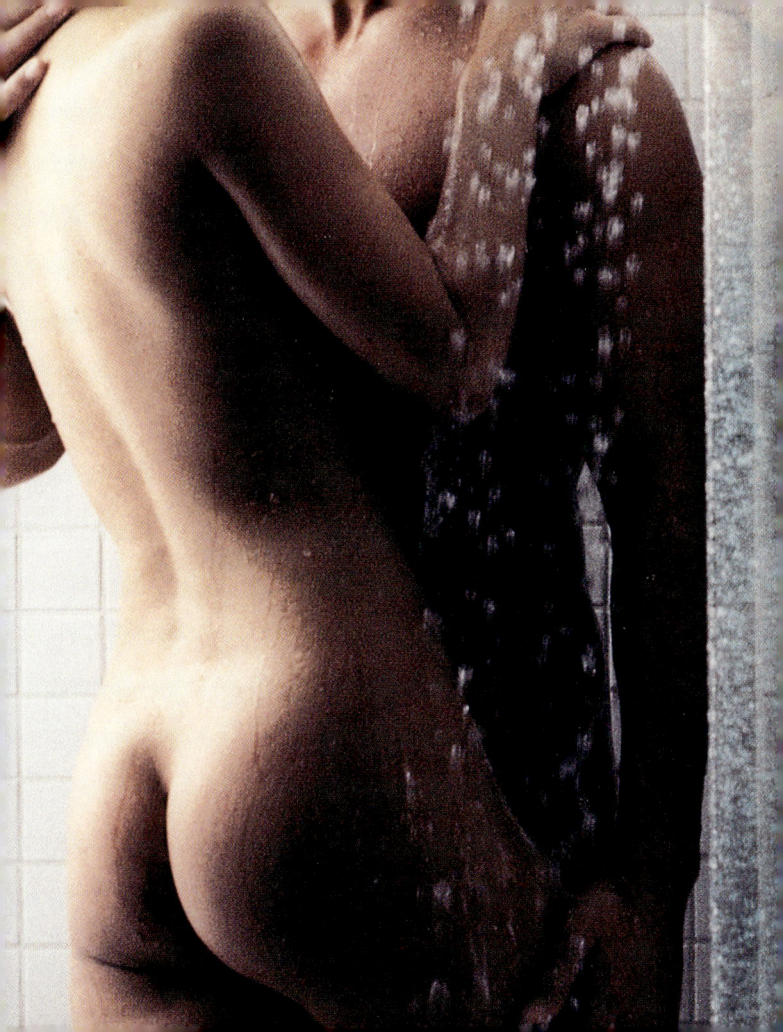

SEX GAMES

NAUGHTY
NEGS

❤ Take saucy photos of each other for fun. Just remember to keep them tame if you're sending them off for commercial processing.

❤ Women: take a picture of yourself dressed up in the style of a vintage pin-up.

❤ Men: take a picture of yourself working out in the gym.

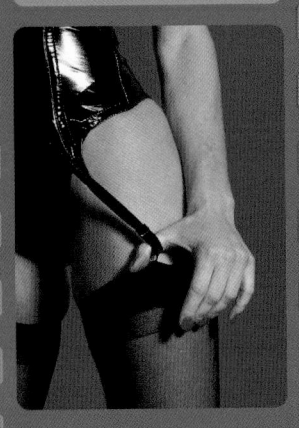

❤ For X-rated pictures, develop your own black and white photos, or use a polaroid camera.

❤ Stage a sexy photoshoot. You're the glamour model. Your lover is the photographer about to lose their professional cool.

❤ Take some artistic shots of each other naked behind glass or in the shower.

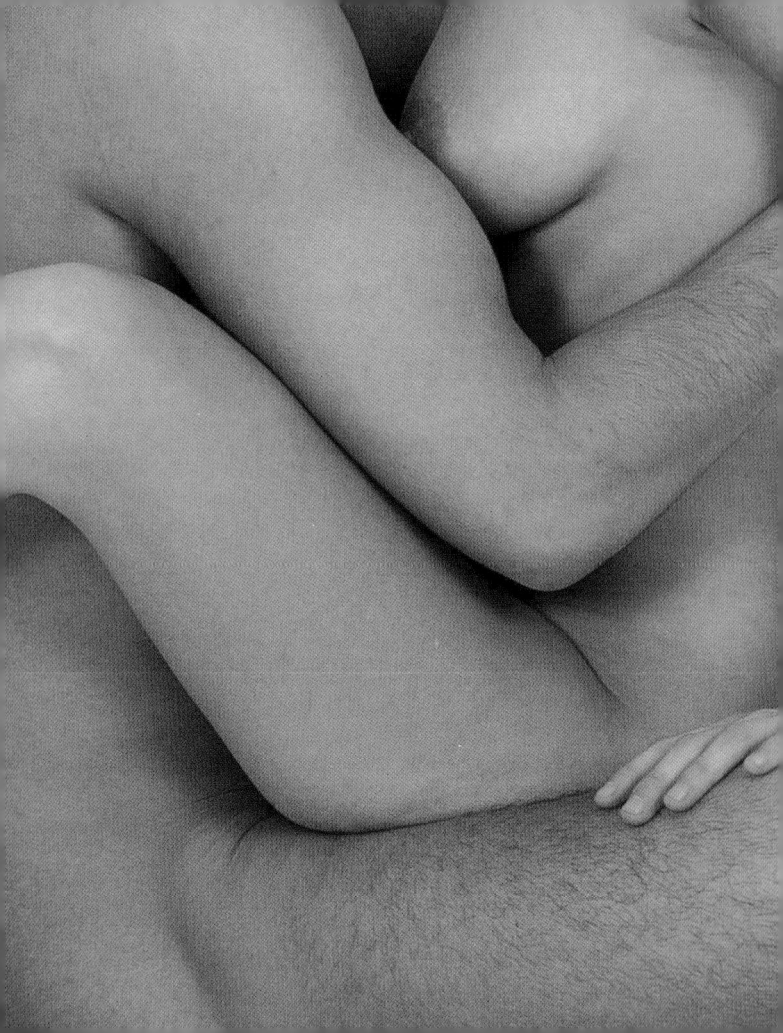

EASTERN EROTICA

❤ The **Kama Sutra** is the best known of the ancient Eastern sex manuals, but also try reading the **Ananga Ranga**, **The Perfumed Garden**, and **The Tao of Sex**.

❤ For something contemporary, try **Zen Sex – The Way of Making Love** by Philip Toshio Sudo, or **Sexual Healing Through Yin and Yang** by Zaihong Shen.

❤ Have an Eastern sex night, when you put some of those exotic positions into practice.

SEX GAMES

GUYS AND GIRLS ON
FILM

❤ Create a special erotic memento in the form of your own personal video. Shoot your partner undressing, or use a camera on a tripod to capture the two of you in action.

❤ If you want something more ambitious, write your own story line and set up the props and location first. You could make the film in the style of your favorite director.

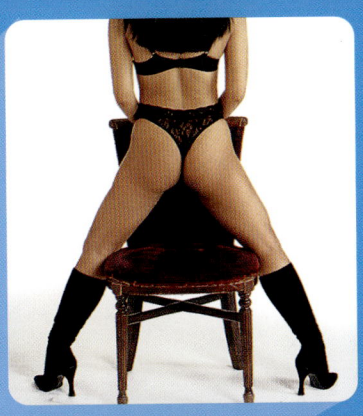

❤ Remember that you can often create a sexy effect by underplaying erotic scenes.

❤ Make different videos with different moods: slow and sensual, or fast and wild, for example.

❤ Be warned – once you're on digital film, you can be beamed around the globe!

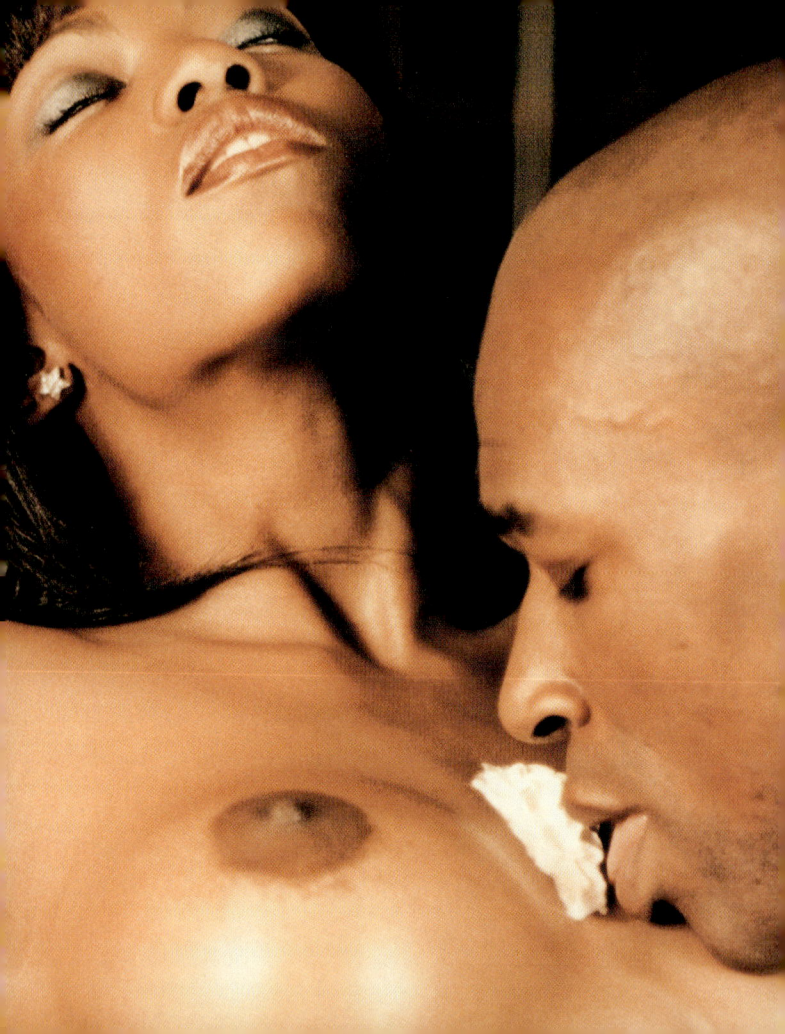

SEX GAMES

ICE-CREAM
CONE

❤ Are you an ice-cream lover? Do you imagine combining your sweet tooth with your other favorite pastime? Is your lover fanatic about the slippery, soft taste of a vanilla cone? If so, have ice-cream sex.

❤ Swirl an icy cone along your lover's body. Circle the nipples, belly, and genitals to create a sweet, shivery trail of pleasure. Now lap it all up with your tongue.

SEX GAMES

SECRET ART

❤ Finding a tattoo unexpectedly on a lover's body always adds an extra buzz to sex. If you don't want the real thing, try surprising your partner with a temporary decoration.

❤ Good tattoo territory is just above the cleft of your buttocks, just below your navel, or on your inner thighs.

SEX GAMES

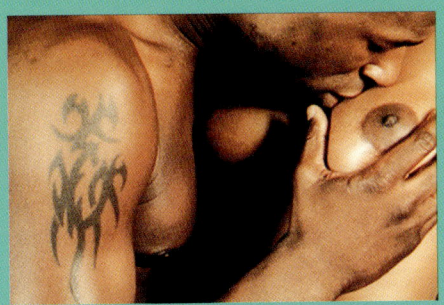

♥ Go out wearing his 'n' hers tattoos.

♥ Write your lover's name somewhere on your body and challenge him to find it.

♥ Write a secret message in mirror writing on your lover's back and tell her to read it later in private.

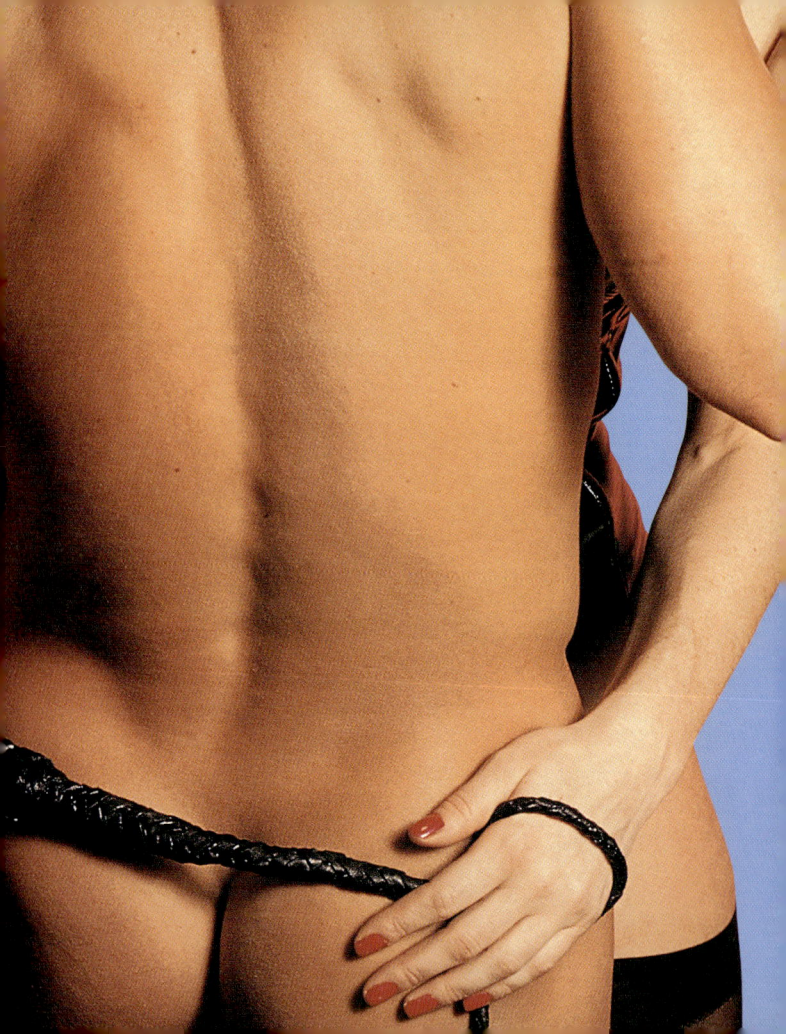

SEX GAMES

GENDER
BENDING

❤ Experiment with gender roles by dressing up as the opposite sex. See what effect this has on your behavior.

❤ Get your partner to do the same. (You can even give each other dress and makeup tips.)

❤ Now try kissing, caressing, and making love in your new roles. Behave as authentically as you can – and then just see what interesting things unfold!

SEX GAMES

SEX
DIARY

❤ Use a notebook to record your sexual dreams, thoughts, and experiences.

❤ If you masturbate to a specific fantasy, write it in your notebook.

❤ Women: note whether or not you feel sexy on each day of the month. This way you can chart the natural peaks and troughs of your sex drive. And then you can act on them!

SEX GAMES

❤ Hold a diary reading evening when your lover gets the chance to hear about the "blue movies of your mind."

❤ Photocopy diary extracts and give them to your lover as a unique sex gift.

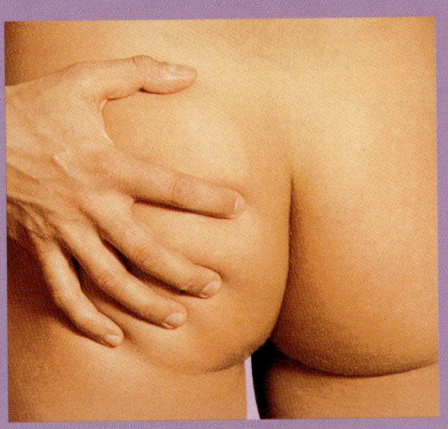

SEX GAMES

MY HANDS ARE
TIED

❤ Your assignment is to make mad, passionate love to your partner without using your hands. This forces you to rely on your arms, lips, tongue, feet, genitals, belly, chest, and nipples – and a lot of imagination!

❤ Tie your lover's hands and then make love to them. This way they have no choice but to give in to sensual pleasure.

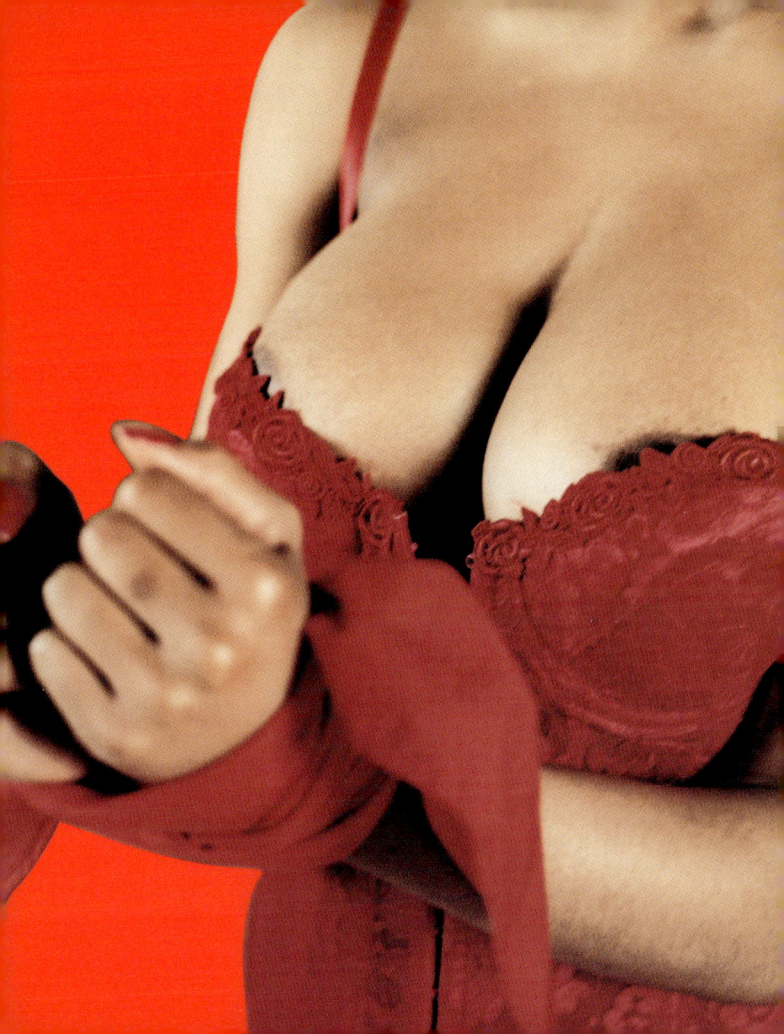

INDEX

A B

Against the wall, sex 144–5
Bathing, oil 68–9
Bathtime sex 8, 58–61
Bedrooms 48–9
Bedtime stories 78–9
Belly 88, 120
Biting 200–1
Blindfolds 130, 160–1, 164–5
Body painting 186–7
Bondage 172–3, 234–5
Boudoirs 48–9
Breasts 56, 75, 131
Buttocks 115, 140, 172–3

C

Cameras 63, 189, 220–1
Caresses 65
Champagne 18, 27, 54
Cleavage caress 110
Clitoris 57, 90, 125, 126–9, 131, 137, 142–3, 150–1

Clothes, sexy 32–3
Condoms 49, 112–3, 159, 183
Cosmetics 36
Costumes 192

D

Diary, sex 232–3
Do-It-Yourself sex 42–3
"Doctors and nurses" games 202–3
Dressing down 20–1
Dressing up 7

E

Eastern erotica 222–3
Edible sex 210–1
Erogenous zones 56–7
Erotic games 190–235
Erotic talk 45
Erotic toys 156–89
Eye contact 25

INDEX

F

Fantasies 190–235
Flirting 22–5
Food, and sex 8, 28–9, 152–3, 155, 184–5, 188–9, 210–3, 226–7

G

G-spot 118–9, 120, 126, 131
Garters 20–1, 53
Gender swapping 230–1

H

Honey 152–3
Honeymoon again 198–9
"Hot and cold" game 120
Hugging 65

I K

Ice-cream 226–7
Ice-cubes 134
Imagination 128–9, 192, 234
In the Mood 38–79
Internet sex 34–5, 158–9
Kissing 40, 200–1

L

Lace 170–1
Leather 169, 173
Legs 32–3
Licking 88–9
Lingerie 27, 159
Lip gloss 17
Lips 17
Loving her 116–155
Loving him 80–115
Lubricants 113, 159

M

Masks 169, 192
Masochism 196–7, 204–5
Massage 51, 90–1, 122–3, 149
Massage oil 48–9, 56, 68–9, 76, 110
Masturbation
  female 42–3, 122–3

INDEX

  male 42–3, 84–5
Mega-orgasm 102
Mirror sex 63
Missionary position 140
Morning sex 109
Mouth 40–1, 87, 109
Movie sex 216–7, 224–5

N

Navel 88
Nipple clamps 115
Nipples 88, 115, 131, 134

O

Oral sex 54, 82–3, 87, 106–7, 126
Orgasm 137, 150–1
  serial 150–1

P

Painting, body 186–7
Peek-a-boo 74–5
Peephole sex 214–5
Penetration, deep 94–7

Penis 56, 84–5, 88, 91, 98, 109, 146–7
Pheromones 14–15
Photographic sex 220–1
Pillow books 6
Prolonging the pleasure 105
Push-ups 140

Q R

Quick sex 93
Relaxation 105
Romance 18–19
Romantic meals 28–9
Rough sex 139
Rubber 166–7

S

Sado-masochism 196–7, 204–5
Saliva 84, 106–7
Satin 170–1
Sauna sex 76–7
Scented oils 48–9, 71
Schoolgirl fantasies 206–7
Seduction 10–37

INDEX

Sensation rating 57
Sensitive spots 115
Sensual smells 71
Sex games 190–235
Sex shops 158–9
Sex standing up 145
Sex talk 45
Sex tokens 30–1
Shower sex 218–19
Silk 20, 178
Smell, sensual 70–1
Solo-style sex 63
Spanking 180–1
Spine tingler 148–9
Spontaneous sex 93
Standing up, sex 145
Stockings 20–1, 53
Striptease 66
Surprises, saucy 27

T U

Tattoos 228–9
Telephone sex 34–5
Tender talk 133
Testicles 82–3
Textures 48–9, 84, 170–1
Thai massage 90–1
Thighs 115
Three-Hander 98
Toes 46
Tongue 46, 125, 126–9
Torso 36
Toy box 160–3
Toys, erotic 156–89
Treasure hunt 194–5
"Truth or dare" game 209
Underwear, rubber 166–7

V

Vagina 98, 100–1, 126, 150
Vaginal grip 100–1
Vegetables 188–9
Vibrators 102, 120, 129, 131, 159, 174–5, 176–7
Visual sex 12

W X Y

Water-based jelly 69
Weekends away 72–3
X-rated positions 146–7
Yogic sex 105

239

ACKNOWLEDGEMENTS

Acknowledgements

For their work on the original edition, DK would like to thank Karen Ward, Senior Art Editor; Stephanie Farrow, Managing Editor; Kesta Desmond, Project Editor; Karen Constanti, DTP; and Joanna Bull, Production.

PHOTOGRAPHY: Luc Beziat; Patricia Morris; James Muldowney. All images © Dorling Kindersley. For further information see: www.dkimages.com.

PROPS: Ann Summers for the loan of lingerie.
Skin Two for the loan of pvc and rubber outfits.
Harmony for the loan of lingerie, pvc outfits, and accessories.

For good quality sex aids try:

UK
Passion8, NES Limited, 4 Kilnbeck Business Park,
Beverley HU17 0LF
Tel: 01482 873377
www.passion8.co.uk

Ann Summers
For your nearest store, or to organize a party, phone 0845 456 2399
or visit www.annsummers.com

Skin Two (for pvc and bondage equipment)
Tel: 020 8208 7955
www.skintwo.com

Harmony
167 Charing Cross Road, London WC2H 0EN,
103 Oxford Street, London W1D 2HF and
4 Walkers Court, London W1R 3FQ
www.harmonyxxx.com

US
Good Vibrations
Retail stores in San Francisco, Berkeley, and Brookline. Online store at www.goodvibes.com
Tel: (415) 974 8985

AUSTRALIA
Sexcitement
A selection of toys, accessories, and clothing.
www.sexcitement.com.au
Email: sales@sexcitement.com.au